MILLION DOLLAR DENTISTRY

*The Astonishing, Proven Way
That Highly Successful Dentists
Manage Their Patients,
Their Teams, and Their Finances*

From the Creator of The NextLevel Practice™

GARY KADI

Million Dollar Dentistry

Million Dollar Dentistry books may be purchased in quantities for educational, business or promotional use. For information go to www.garykadi.com.

ISBN: 978-0-9820719-1-5

Fifth Edition
Printed on acid-free paper

Acknowledgments

To my clients: Thank you for your trust and the privilege of working with you. I know it takes a lot to allow a person into one of your most valued possessions, and I do not take our relationship lightly.

To my many mentors and manuscript readers: Thank you for your time, insight, and candor, which make this book even more valuable and easier to read and understand.

To my friend Michael Levin: Thank you for your ability to turn a great book into an I-cannot-put-this-book-down-until-I'm-finished book.

To my friend Michael Fishman: Thank you for your limitless contribution and generous giving to my work and life. To my amazing Team: Thank you for the world class difference you make in the lives of every person you touch. You are world class and you are the change you wish to see in the world.

To my best friend and dear wife, Judith: Thank you from the bottom of my heart for your unconditional loving support and the birth of Rome Jacob. I admire and appreciate your beauty, grace, and love. I am completely honored to be your husband.

To my son, Rome: Thank you for the true joy of being your father. You have taken me beyond my reality of love.

To my family: Thank you for instilling great values in me and for your unconditional love and support.

Personal Insights
and Reader Feedback
Since the First Edition

T O PUT IT SIMPLY, dentistry rocks. The current boom in dentistry, combined with the desire of dentists to make their practices more successful than ever, has created a huge response to this book. That response took us to our second printing only five months after the book was published. I am now proud to offer this updated version of *Million Dollar Dentistry*, complete with a number of new thoughts and insights. These insights occurred largely as the result of comments from many of our readers, and also from my own experiences as I seek to live the concepts in the book. (Yes, I practice what I preach!)

With expansion in the dental marketplace and a larger need for dental care, the treatment commonly delivered to clients typically fails to live up to the comprehensive care dental teams seek to provide. Most practices want to provide quality quadrant care, but the majority of teams are frustrated by their patients' resistance and unwillingness to accept and pay for that kind of full treatment. This frustration commonly starts in the thought pattern held by a majority of dental teams—they believe that most patients cannot afford complete care. It's the experience of many teams that patients seek care only when notable and persistent pain occurs.

We take a different position. By establishing a proactive approach, it's possible to offset these beliefs and behaviors, resulting in patients receiving all the care they need. Instead of complaining about the price or complaining over the bill, patients will happily buy your dentistry because they feel educated and in control.

This book addresses these topics and many more. As you read, you'll notice that the subject matter goes way beyond developing skills for managing an efficient practice or developing a stronger bonus system. Those goals merely provide a means to an end. I'll certainly address their importance, but you'll be learning how to build a successful practice at every level. Our goal is to arm you with tools of empowerment that will allow you to become amazingly successful—successful in every part of your life.

This success has the power to completely reshape and redefine your life. It will afford you the ability to travel around the world, purchase the house of your dreams, and have everything you've ever wanted without holding back. And that kind of success comes from only one place: you.

This book will help you regain control of your practice, put solid systems in place, create a good team, play a big game, incorporate good structures, and learn to trust that doubling or tripling your practice is absolutely possible. As you learn the NextLevel Methodology™, you will gain applicable tools, resources, and systems, in addition to developing a mindset of abundance. With this new, limitless attitude, you'll put into practice the philosophy of "having it all," which means generating more money while creating the time and freedom to enjoy it. Imagine your life with more freedom, reduced stress, a happy team, patients who comply, and more money than you need. That's the life I envision for you. And with the help of this book, that's the life you can have.

Million Dollar Dentistry unveils the powerful NextLevel Methodology™. For more than a decade, I've enjoyed working with many private clients who have been reaping the benefits of this system for some time. Now I'm introducing the methodology to the public. This book resulted from many years of research, refinement, testing, and requests from my clients to codify and capture the unique tenets of my methodology. Through reading this book, you'll gain a taste of what NextLevel represents and how it has produced exponential success for my clients. My system simplifies practice management and reassigns control to the dentist. At the core, it offers a unique triple-win system, which provides substantial benefits to the doctor, the office team, and the patient. The triple-win system practically self-renews; once fully implemented, it manages itself with only modest attention.

I hope that by reading this book, you will absorb and apply some of these formulas to your own practice. I encourage you to pull every grain of inspiration from these pages that could possibly help your practice. Apply it. Use it. And even if, after reading the entire book, you apply just one of these lessons to your practice, you will see extraordinary results. The triple-win concept rewards dentists with improved income, unlimited freedom, and an enhanced lifestyle. Team members become more motivated and attentive as they participate and share in the success of the practice. And patients respond enthusiastically as they receive complete, impeccable care.

Part of our system involves addressing the patient's concern through education, which serves to identify and neutralize their fears. Patients whose fears have been addressed are significantly more likely to commit to complete dental care—not only essential treatment and preventative care, but cosmetic treatment as well.

We also help dentists find a new way to play the "mental game" by demonstrating how to think about your practice so that you maximize your effectiveness and your income. I have no doubt that you'll find the comprehensive strategy and unique philosophy that underlie the NextLevel Methodology™ fascinating. As you'll see, our system consists of practical applications and methods used and tested in practices throughout the country.

And it really works! Our clients who work directly with us often report an increase of 50 percent in revenues. Most report that they double or triple their income. With our help, you can achieve the same level of success. We believe so strongly in our methods that we guarantee serious results.

This book is an introduction to these methods. It will open your mind, enabling you and your team to overcome any philosophical, mental, or emotional biases that could be prohibiting your unlimited success. The systems and tools inside this book will help you create a growing and profitable practice.

If after reading *Million Dollar Dentistry*, you are aligned with this methodology and want support in reaching your own personal next level, the following steps will help you get there:

1.   Read my articles at www.GaryKadi.com/dental_industry_articles.html.

2.   Call my office for a complimentary 30-minute consultation with me at 866-926-0914.

I wish you the very best success.

Gary Kadi
Scottsdale, Arizona

Contents

Chapter 1

A Day in the Life of
Larry Laserguy, D.D.S.

Monday morning.

THE TWO MOST DREADED words in the life of Larry Laserguy, D.D.S.

As he piloted his newly leased 7 Series BMW from his multimillion-dollar home in the best neighborhood in town to his ultramodern suite of dental offices in the best medical building in the region, his life somehow made no sense to him.

A highly successful dentist with twenty years of experience; a large, thriving and lucrative practice; a gorgeous second wife and three attractive, athletic and capable kids, Larry felt as though he should have been on Cloud Nine. Instead, the only numbers that formed in his mind were 911. His life felt like an ongoing emergency, and no one was there to answer the call.

As he navigated the early morning traffic, sipping on his Starbucks and glancing at his new Rolex—a gift from his wife, although it was a gift that he would ultimately pay for, since he was the sole provider—Larry felt that nagging sense of upset in the pit of his stomach. The Monday morning team meeting, to begin in fifteen minutes, should be a weekly cause for celebration. After all, the office was jammed with patients, new and old. A sense of what Larry liked to call "organized chaos" pervaded the entire practice, giving off a sense of importance and success. Every year, the office grossed more and more money, enrolled more new patients, closed more cases. Larry's bi-monthly draw represented far more money than he ever expected to make. It was certainly radically more money than his father had ever made, and yet his father had paid off their house early, bought all of his new cars for cash, and sent Larry and his brother and sister to private colleges and to dental, medical, and law school, without benefit of scholarships.

And his father had never even been to college.

As Larry's beautiful office tower came into view, he thought for a brief moment about how the weekend had gone. It had gone badly. He and his wife, Linda, had had one of those big blowups—over money, as usual. The kids, all in their teens, were expecting new cars for their birthdays, the kinds of cars that they could drive with pride at their private high schools and private colleges. The cost of insuring three teenagers on the road—he'd just gotten a quote from his insurance buddy at the club—made Larry just shake his head. And they couldn't have driven ten-year-old clunkers, the kind that Larry drove all through college and dental school. No way. For Larry's kids, even a 3 Series BMW was a compromise, and not a happy one at that.

They also had fought again about the idea of installing a home theater, something Linda wanted to begin immediately. After all, half a dozen families in their gated community already had home theaters installed, and Linda didn't want to feel as if their family were being left behind. The idea was enticing to Larry, who imagined himself on a Sunday afternoon watching an NFL game with half a dozen of his envious buddies, reclining on buttery leather seats in front of a screen the size of which you would expect to see in a cineplex. Talk about looking like you've arrived.

But arrived where? The poorhouse? The only downside with the home theater was the price. Larry's parents' first (and only) house had cost less than the estimate that the guy from the home theater company had presented. But Linda was digging in her heels; she really wanted it, and he did not want to let her down.

With interest rates ticking upward, payments on the interest only adjustable-rate super jumbo mortgage and the second mortgage were steadily, ominously creeping up, and Larry had the sneaking feeling that not only was he building no equity, he was actually going backwards. Just last night, Larry had checked his bank balance before he went to bed—always a bad idea—only to discover that he was overdrawn, again, this time to the tune of $4,300. And yet Linda still wanted to install that home theater and buy all the kids new cars. Yikes.

Larry pulled into his reserved parking space and put on his game face, ready to start the new day. Maybe the Monday morning team meeting would go well, for a change.

But as Larry rode the elevator to his top-floor office, with its commanding view of the city, he knew it wouldn't.

"Good morning, Doctor Laserguy." Diane, his trusted office manager of nineteen years, greeted him with a smile as he stepped into the office. "How was your weekend?"

"Fine," Larry lied. As usual, Larry was a bit too consumed with his own concerns to ask Diane how her weekend went; he gave no indication that he noticed the slight frown on her face due to his perpetual neglect of her emotional well-being. Larry knew well, nonetheless, that Diane was the linchpin of his entire organization. Without her, he knew well, his practice would implode. When she took her annual vacation, two weeks that filled Larry's every waking thought for the preceding two months with dread, he typically ended up doing the million and one things that Diane did. She did them cheerfully, gracefully, and always with a smile. He did them reluctantly, unhappily, and in stark terror that he was going to run out of time. He knew Diane had been entertaining offers from other dental practices, and he had had no choice but to constantly raise her salary. Diane now made a very nice living as an office manager. And unlike Larry, when she had a paycheck, she cashed it immediately.

Larry's paychecks, large as they were, would ride around in his wallet for weeks, sometimes for a month or more, until those rare, blissful moments of cash flow that permitted him to actually deposit the darned things.

Even at that moment, Larry could feel the weight of two paychecks in his pocket, his compensation for the last two pay periods, totaling almost $30,000. That money would go a long way toward resolving the overdraft, taking care of his mortgage payment, and putting down a down payment on the home theater, which Linda would not be denied, and which he really wanted as much as she did. But Larry had somehow developed the philosophy of "pay yourself last," simply because if he didn't pay everybody else, and if he didn't pay his vendors, nobody would show up at his office.

If he didn't cash those paychecks, his accountant had warned him, he would be late—again—on his mortgage, and his formerly pristine, 800+ credit score would slip a tiny bit further.

Larry shook his head quickly, as if to banish all thoughts of personal and business finance, and he strode purposefully toward the conference room for the team meeting.

Larry believed in starting team meetings promptly, at exactly 7:30 a.m. Larry was the only person on his team who felt that way. Everybody else straggled in between 7:30 and 7:40, to Larry's weekly consternation, chatting about the weekend bachelorette party in Vegas that two of them had attended and little Jimmy's soccer game and the other sorts of things that people talk about as they gather on Monday mornings in workplaces everywhere.

Larry took their lateness and their lack of desire to focus on the important matters at hand as a personal affront. Larry vaguely sensed that his team, for all the salary and benefits he provided them, didn't like him, and this fact pained him. He didn't understand why they didn't like him. He was as competent as any dentist in the city, he never fired anybody, and his salary and benefits package was comparable to most of the other dental practices around town. Sure, some people paid more, but Larry believed in frugality, especially when it came to paying salaries. Thirteen dollars an hour was plenty, especially when given the attitude of the kinds of people who came to work in dental offices, Larry believed.

It was 7:35 before enough people were present for the meeting to begin. Larry's partner, Charlie Chairside, D.M.D., was nowhere to be seen. He typically made a grand entrance about ten minutes into the meeting. What was *with* that guy, Larry thought, as he surveyed his unruly troops. How does he manage to close cases with just about everybody who walks into his office, while I struggle to close one-third of the people I talk to? And why does he think he's so important that he can just walk into an all-hands meeting whenever he wants? Exactly what kind of example is he setting for everyone else?

At that exact moment, Charlie strode in, flashing his movie star smile at the assembled throng—the dental hygienists, the front desk people, the assistants, the whole team. As soon as Charlie came in, a hush fell over the group, and they all turned expectantly toward Diane to find out what was going on.

Why does he get more respect than I do? Larry asked himself, and then he turned to Diane and said, as he did every Monday morning, "How do we look?"

Diane grimaced and tried to cover it quickly with a smile, but everybody could tell that it was going to be another crazy Monday morning.

"Here we go," Diane began, reading from her handwritten notes. "We're packed today, and we have six emergencies. I hope you all have your roller skates on."

A general groan went up from the group.

"Good old Ms. Backbreaker is scheduled for her fifth redo on number nineteen," she said, as Larry rolled his eyes. "She's scheduled for four units and I only need fifteen minutes."

Larry looked heavenwards and asked silently, why me? Ms. Backbreaker was never satisfied with his work and, for that matter, never paid for it, either. She must owe the office thousands. Probably exactly as much as I'm overdrawn at the bank.

"WE'RE PACKED TODAY, AND WE HAVE SIX EMERGENCIES. I HOPE YOU ALL HAVE YOUR ROLLER SKATES ON."

Anita, the appointment coordinator, gave Diane something of an angry look. "Yeah," Anita said, her jaw tense. "But you talk to her for fifteen and you take calls for fifteen and then you hang out at your desk for fifteen."

Larry didn't want this weekly meeting to dissolve into arguments, as they often did. "We need to talk about scheduling at our next team meeting," Larry said. "Let's not waste time. What else is happening, Diane?"

"Jennifer Hanson is coming in at 11:00," she said, looking at her notes. "But the case is not back from the lab. And by the way, does anybody know where Amy is? The new lab coordinator?"

Dani, one of the hygienists, spoke up. "She's out today," Dani said. "She called this morning and sounded terrible."

Larry sighed. "Diane," he said, "see me after this meeting regarding Amy. And call the lab immediately."

Diane nodded. "Okay," she said. "Let's move on. Our daily goal, as you all know, is $10,000. Unfortunately, we've only got $3,200 on the books, and five hygiene patients cancelled. We need the hygienists to get on the phone and fill their schedules. Okay?"

Suzi and Dani, the dental hygienists, rolled their eyes. Like most dental hygienists, they believed that their jobs were to clean teeth—not to support the re-care system, call old patients, educate the patients they do see about cosmetic dentistry, answer the phones, close cases, propose dental work, or do any of the myriad things that Larry kept telling them to do.

Larry could never understand the star mentality that dental hygienists possessed. After all, what exactly was so glamorous about cleaning teeth all day long? Where did they get so much attitude from? You'd think they were all in Hollywood, getting ready for their starring roles, the way they carried on. Larry watched Dani and Suzi's body language. You could see that if they didn't have any patients, they were going to sit around and make phone calls to friends, get their nails done, or do anything other than something that might be useful and productive for the office. Obviously not team players.

I'd fire them in a heartbeat, Larry thought, if they weren't so good-looking.

At that moment, Denise, the one staff member who stayed outside the meeting and handled incoming calls, stuck her head in the door.

"Dr. Laserguy," she said urgently, "your wife, your lawyer, and the home theater guy are holding for you, and your eight o'clock is seated in room three. And you got an e-mail from the bank about your—"

"I know all about it," Larry said quickly, embarrassed to have his personal finances a potential topic of discussion at the team meeting. What a great way to start the day, he thought.

"Tell them all I'll call them back."

"Your wife is insisting," Denise said, with that look in her eye that suggested that Larry better take the call.

"Tell her to hold a little longer," Larry said wearily. "I'll be right there." He turned back to the group. "Anything else?" he asked, anxious to get the call with Linda over with so he could finally get chairside in room three.

"Mary, the new dental assistant?" Diane said, her voice rising an octave as she spoke, as if she were asking a question.

"What about her?" Larry growled. A more incompetent assistant he had never seen in his entire life. He'd forgotten all about Mary, with everything else on his mind. Another day with Mary was positively going to drive him nuts, maybe drive him out of dentistry altogether.

"She quit," Diane said. "She called me over the weekend."

"But why?" Larry asked, stunned. "Do we have anybody to replace her?"

"She said that you yelled at her in front of a patient." And there was general tittering among the office team. Larry, truth be told, had a reputation for speaking sharply to team members in front of the patients.

Well, why not? He was a perfectionist, and he wanted to do perfect dental work. And if the team members couldn't keep up with him or do things the right way the first time, that was their problem, not his. He was the commander in chief, and the chair was his operating theater. And anybody who couldn't hang with that was welcome to hit the trail.

"I couldn't find anybody on such short notice," Diane said, embarrassed. "She called me late last night. She also said that she was talking to a lawyer. Something about sexual harassment, Dr. Laserguy?"

Charlie Chairside looked up quickly from his Blackberry. Larry reddened. He'd made a few innocent jokes to Mary, who really was very attractive. An *attorney*? Didn't anybody have a sense of humor anymore?

"Anything else?" he sighed.

"Just a couple of more things," Diane said, and from the expression on her face, they didn't look like positive things. Larry glanced at his partner, Charlie, who had gone back to his Blackberry and was doing his e-mail and checking his portfolio in front of everybody. Charlie wasn't even paying attention! What kind of team player was he?

"Julie, the insurance coordinator?" Diane began. "Well, she opened the supply closet, and it was jammed so tight with all kinds of junk that a computer monitor fell on her toes. She was wearing sandals, and she thinks she broke a couple of toes."

"Oh, no," Larry muttered, wishing that he could magically vanish from the team meeting and head to the only place in the world where he truly felt safe and in control— next to his chair, alongside a patient.

"And the Jerome family is coming in later today," Diane added, avoiding looking at her boss while she mentioned the name of the family the whole office called the Dental Deadbeats. "They still owe $2475 on their account, and they're only paying fifteen dollars a month. Are you sure you still want to treat them?"

"Who's in charge," Larry asked, looking around the room, "of managing our accounts, so that we don't have situations like this?"

Everybody looked at the floor. Nobody was in charge, Larry realized. We'd better get this handled, he thought. We just can't go on like this.

"Anything else?" he said, feeling emotionally drained. And it wasn't even 7:45 yet. Denise stuck her head in the door and gave Larry another anxious look. Obviously, his wife, his lawyer, and his home theater guy were all still holding. And before long he'd be chairside with the Jerome family, the most phobic group of gaggers and squirmers he had ever seen in his entire career.

There's got to be a better way, Larry said to himself, as he adjourned the meeting and went to take the calls from the three people he wanted to speak to the least at that moment. There's got to be a better way.

If anything of the foregoing sounds in any way familiar to you, you're not alone. I consult to dentists across the country who face, to varying degrees, the problems of Larry Laserguy—problems that threaten to swamp or even destroy dental practices, problems that lead to financial disaster, broken marriages, unhappy relationships with children, and the sort of ongoing misery that countless highly successful dentists face and have no one with whom they can discuss it.

The sad truth is that countless dentists deal with many of these problems every single day of their lives. They're frustrated, they're angry, and they've got no idea what to do. They need a break, and they need someone who understands. Most of all, they need solutions.

Larry's story, as comical as it might be to somebody who isn't undergoing all these multiple crises, admittedly is an exaggeration of the problems dentists face. Yes, many dentists generate huge amounts of income in their highly successful practices, but their expenses, at home and at work, are even greater. I work with some dentists who have been practicing for decades and have nothing to show for it but six- and even seven-figure levels of debt.

They sense that their team members dislike them and sometimes even hate them and that their partners disrespect them, and they cannot figure out why. They are happiest chairside yet find themselves performing the sorts of management and office tasks that they cannot understand why their team doesn't have the common sense or even the decency to handle. After all, that's what they're getting paid for.

It gets worse. They have patients who drive them crazy, who don't pay, who cancel with no notice, and who generally make their lives miserable. They have ongoing cash flow crises that turn their entire business and personal financial lives into houses of cards. And they feel that there is no end in sight.

These dentists pay me six figures to solve these and similar problems. My promise to them—which I back up with a one hundred percent guarantee—is that I will work with them to show them how to solve their problems and enjoy a guaranteed minimum of a dollar-for-dollar return on investment for my services. The average office increases collections twenty to fifty percent in the first year, and income continues to grow year after year. My clients describe the residual effect of my work as an annuity: the increases in income, happiness, and peace of mind that ratchet up every single year.

Your business becomes your best possible investment— it becomes much more prudent for you to invest in your own business than in anyone else's on the stock market, where you're not in control.

MY CLIENTS DESCRIBE THE RESIDUAL EFFECT OF MY WORK AS AN ANNUITY— THE INCREASES IN INCOME, HAPPINESS, AND PEACE OF MIND RATCHET UP EVERY SINGLE YEAR.

In this book, I'm going to share with you the solutions that I implement with my clients, who resolve their debt crises, their staffing crises, and their marital and family crises. They also end up with far more money in the pocket, far more time chairside relative to other tasks, and far more career and life satisfaction and happiness than they ever dreamt was possible. I help these dentists lead the lives that they are entitled to enjoy, after all the hard work they have put into their training and after the years of work they have put into building their practices.

This is not a book about how to start a dental

practice—you could find plenty of those. And this is not cookie-cutter consulting that doesn't grasp the real dilemmas dentists face. Instead, together, we are going to expose—and solve—the kinds of problems that dentists face that nobody wants to talk about and that very few people know how to solve. I know how to solve these problems. I've done it for countless dentists, and together, I'm going to do the same thing for you.

The scenario we just viewed, that of Larry Laserguy and his mounting personal, financial, and professional woes, paints a picture of the extreme situations in which many of my clients find themselves before they come to me. In the next chapter, I'd like to paint a very different picture for you. I'd like to show you the life that you are entitled to lead, and just how much joy, excitement, and success you can reap. And I'll show you how to work less and make more money, too. So let's take a look right now at the life you deserve to live, and let's find out together exactly how to make it a reality for you.

Take Your Practice to the NextLevel:

1. Many highly successful dentists lead a double life. Their world sees them as affluent and powerful, but in reality they are struggling to maintain control over their financial situations and their teams.

    Look at your life and make a list of all the things you don't want other people to know about you. What are you withholding? What are you not saying that needs to be said? Making this list will help you identify the parts of your life that could use a jolt of authenticity, responsibility and communication.

2. I've worked with dentists for long enough to recognize the specific problems they face—at the office, with their teams, with their patients, with their spouses and children, and in their financial lives. That's why my methodology is designed to address the dentist's unique plight.

3. Even highly successful dentists can find new levels of professional satisfaction and financial success… if they only know how.

Chapter 2

The Life You are Entitled to Lead

IN THE PREVIOUS CHAPTER, I painted a fairly bleak, if all too accurate, picture of what many dentists' lives resemble—an outward display of success masking a painful sense of desperation fueled by crises at work, at home, and in their financial lives.

It doesn't have to be that way.

In this chapter, I'd like to focus on the sorts of results that my clients have achieved. They now enjoy unimagined financial success. They spend fewer hours at work. They report a much higher degree of job satisfaction, harmony in the workplace (it can happen!) and at home. They even possess a plan for an orderly and well-crafted retirement, so they can do the other things in life that matter to them.

Now it's your turn to live this way.

Throughout the rest of the book, I'll show you how you can achieve each of these goals in your own practice, and I'll show you specific tools, methods, and approaches that have had wonderful, long-lasting results on the bottom line and on the personal satisfaction of my dentist clients. But first, let's paint a picture of exactly how life can be.

Before we get into the specifics of how to achieve these results, let's first talk about what you can reasonably hope to achieve if you are willing to expand your sense of possibility and try a few new approaches to the practice—and the business—of dentistry.

1. Have All the Income You Desire.

Before anything else, I get my clients to dream big dreams. As the expression says, "Green goes with everything." There's nothing like a healthy, regular dose of high income to make people feel good about themselves, their dental practice, and their personal lives. Typically, sole practitioners working with two hygienists in an office gross about $50,000 a month when they come to see me. By implementing the suggestions I offer, they go up to $85,000 a month within the first year, and they continue to achieve similar rates of increase year after year.

BEFORE ANYTHING ELSE, I GET MY CLIENTS TO DREAM BIG DREAMS.

Two dentists working together and employing three dental hygienists typically gross $100,000 a month. My consulting methods take them to a gross of $150,000 per month, and again, the increases keep on coming, year after year.

Three dentists working together and employing five hygienists will typically gross $150,000 a month. I generally take them to between $235,000 and $250,000 a month in gross income.

In the overwhelming majority of cases, my clients achieve these remarkable growth rates *without* adding to their existing team, *without* working additional hours, and without any new forms of marketing. They don't achieve these results with smoke and mirrors. Instead, I show them how to apply the sorts of business practices that simply aren't taught in dental school or, for that matter, anywhere else.

My consulting work typically leads dentists to have a brand new problem—what to do with all the money that's rolling in, far more money than they ever expected to handle. After all, where do you put all that new-found cash that flows in, unceasingly, steadily, month after month, year after year?

That's *exactly* the sort of problem that I want to create for you.

Dentists typically have what I call blind spots in their belief systems. They have caps on what they think they can earn. They don't realize that a well-managed dental office permits a dentist to gross up to a thousand dollars an hour for his or her time chairside. They don't realize that every aspect of their business can be turned into a profit center until I show them exactly how. I'll show you exactly those same methods in this book.

I start off by asking dentists exactly how much money they would *like* to earn. Then I ask them how much money they can earn per hour if the practice is managed well, and then we multiply that figure by the number of hours they wish to work. In so doing, my clients set income goals—often for the first time in their entire careers—and these goals far exceed what they are currently earning.

They have trouble at first believing that they can reach those goals without adding a new team, without working more hours, and without marketing efforts that they fear would make them look unprofessional in their own eyes, in the eyes of their peers, and in the eyes of the general public. But it's entirely possible for a dentist to earn up to a thousand dollars an hour for every hour he practices dentistry. I've shown my clients how to do it, and now it's your turn to have all the income you desire.

2. Work as Many or as Few Hours as You Would Like.

There are three basic ways for dentists to increase production. The first method is that they can increase the number of hours they practice, doing the same amount of production per hour. I don't recommend this method, yet this is the most commonly accepted way for a dentist to make more money.

The second way: Dentists can increase their production per hour, and I show my clients how to do that. Often, my clients find themselves strapped for time and for cash flow. They feel that they are on an endless treadmill, spinning faster and faster, and they are working more and more hours, but they seem to be standing still nonetheless in terms of cash flow and net worth.

Again, it doesn't have to be that way. My clients learn how to increase their productivity per hour and thus reduce the number of hours they work, from thirty-two down to twenty-five, without evenings or weekends. This way, they alleviate the frustration of not being able to spend enough time with their spouses and children. They eliminate the sense of exhaustion and frustration that overwork typically creates. And they have a hell of a lot more fun, too.

The third way to increase income is to increase production and hire an associate at the same time. The new business skills that you will bring to your practice, the second dentist's production, and the equity of his buy-in will combine to radically increase your income. I'll show you how to do all that. The bottom line here: you can work as many or as few hours as you would like, if you know the secrets my clients know about how to increase your production and make each hour spent practicing dentistry truly count.

3. Have Your Patients Show Up—and Have Them Show Up on Time.

One of the most frustrating things about practicing dentistry is that none of your patients want to come see you. They show up late. They cancel appointments at the last minute. Sometimes they don't even give you the courtesy of any notice at all. They back away from the suggestions that you have made about the kind of dental care they need. While you think they have accepted the case you have presented, the reality is that they have no intention at all of letting you do your job.

My clients experienced the frustration I've just described until I taught them methods for educating new patients from the start about the nature of the dental work they truly needed and also *the importance of keeping their commitments.* Believe it or not, there are proven ways to get patients to show up—and show up on time! Imagine how much freer your life would feel if you did not have the constant, nagging irritation of knowing that on any given day some of your patients were bound to cancel the appointments they had made with you, and thus deprive themselves of the dental work they need and deprive you of the income that you deserve.

BELIEVE IT OR NOT, THERE ARE PROVEN WAYS TO GET PATIENTS TO SHOW UP AND SHOW UP ON TIME!

It *is* possible to create a new framework with your patients that has them showing up—and showing up on time—for their dental work.

4. **Be Free to Present Comprehensive Treatment Without Any Fear of Rejection or Negative Reaction from the Patient.**

We all hate rejection, whether in our personal lives or in our professional lives. For dentists, that fear of rejection translates into a myriad of lost opportunities—and lost income. They are trapped by their fear and unable to present the comprehensive treatment that they know their patients need. Dentists are not really doing their patients a service by minimizing real problems, simply because they sense that the patient might say no to comprehensive treatment, might claim to be unable to afford such treatment, or simply won't come back.

In our society, for some bizarre reason, there is a stigma attached to anything to do with sales. Dentists rightly think of themselves as highly educated and highly competent medical professionals. But the reality is that if your office doesn't sell, you can't practice dentistry.

Most dentists are frustrated by the fact that their lives seem to be an endless, boring succession of "drilling, filling, and billing." In other words, they see themselves doing the same relatively dull, mundane tasks of dentistry over and over again, simply because they don't have the selling training necessary to explain to patients what is truly necessary for their optimal dental health. I'm not talking about offering you high pressure sales tactics or sleazy "can't miss" closes. Instead, I'm talking about knowing how to sell in a sophisticated, confident, trustworthy manner that enhances the patient's confidence in you as you accomplish your goal of providing maximum service to your patient.

With the kind of sales techniques I will show you, everybody wins: the patient will get all of the dental care he or she needs, and you will earn more and practice the more interesting kinds of dentistry, the sorts of treatments that require multiple visits, that challenge you and get you out of that "drill, fill, and bill" mentality.

My clients are not afraid to present a comprehensive case and complex cases, and they thoroughly enjoy the process. And their confidence in the ability of the entire team to sell cases has a huge impact both on the dental health of their patients and on their own financial bottom line.

5. Have Patients Accept at Least Eighty Percent of Treatment Presented and Pay For It... in Full and in Advance.

These must seem like outrageous claims to the average dentist who struggles to convince patients to accept anything more complicated than a couple of fillings. The fact is that if you present a case properly, you have every reason to expect that your patient will accept that case eighty percent of the time. Not only that, I will show you how to have your patient pay in full for that treatment—and pay in advance.

Most dentists look inside the patient's mouth and present the solution—you need three crowns, you need a bridge, whatever. The acceptance rate for dentists who practice in this traditional manner, I have discovered, is approximately thirty-eight percent. In other words, in most offices, patients are rejecting their dentists' recommendations almost two-thirds of the time. Actually, most dentists don't even track this figure, and they are often quite surprised to learn just how low their acceptance rate really is. Why is the rate traditionally so low? It's because these dentists only present solutions.

Your patient will accept treatment far more often if you also present the problem in all its clarity by use of an intraoral camera, so that you show the patient exactly what has to be treated. On top of that, I can show you how to explain to the patient exactly what the dream of one hundred percent dental health looks like. When you combine these three elements—the problem, the solution, and the implications for complete dental health—your closing rate will shoot up, just as my clients have experienced.

> **WHEN YOU COMBINE THESE THREE ELEMENTS—THE PROBLEM, THE SOLUTION, AND THE IMPLICATIONS FOR COMPLETE DENTAL HEALTH —YOUR CLOSING RATE WILL SHOOT UP, JUST AS MY CLIENTS HAVE EXPERIENCED.**

6. See the Exact Type of Patient You Enjoy Seeing and Do the Exact Type of Dentistry You Want to Do.

These concepts tie in with the points we discussed earlier— the idea that most dentists want to get away from "drilling, filling, and billing." Many dentists have specific types of dentistry that they would prefer to perform. But they can't seem to find patients who need that kind of work or will accept those treatments. These dentists believe patients who can and will accept those kinds of treatments can be found only by resorting to hope and prayer… and external marketing.

Hope and prayer are simply not adequate foundations for building a thriving and lucrative dental practice, as many of my clients had already discovered by the time they came to see me. The fact is that you can perform the kind of dentistry you prefer, and you can find—and sell—the kind of patients to which you aspire, if you only know how. And, as I'm sure you've guessed, I can show you exactly how to find them. Actually, you'll discover that the greatest source of ideal patients… is your appointment book! I'll show you a new way to relate to and care for your current patients that will allow you to do the dentistry you want to do the most.

7. See as Few or as Many Patients as You Would Like.

My clients no longer practice what I call "assembly line" dentistry. They are not tied to finding patient after patient after patient who for the most part can only be sold on the simplest, least lucrative, and least interesting forms of dental care. The key for my clients to moving beyond assembly line dentistry is to understand *how to structure payment schedules.*

This may seem counterintuitive—what exactly do methods of payment have to do with the number of patients you see? The surprising answer is that when you know exactly what payment options to offer—and when to offer them in the selling process—you can sell more people on more care that they truly need.

Let me offer you a different way to think about this issue. Who spends more on a meal in a restaurant—an individual who orders *a la carte*, or someone who orders a *prix fixe* menu? Naturally, it's the person who orders the complete meal. That person knows exactly how much he or she is going to pay for the entire dinner and doesn't leave until the last course is served!

The analogy fits well with the practice of dentistry. Most dentists sell their patients dental services on an *a la carte* basis. It stands to reason that if a dentist knew how to propose and sell patients on *prix fixe* dentistry, that dentist would make far more money than one who continued to offer services *a la carte*. This may seem like an impossible dream for many dentists, but *my* clients do it with ease. They also understand how to remove the question of financing dental treatment from the patient's decision to go ahead with comprehensive treatment. By taking money off the table as an issue, my clients are able to sell far more cases than they ever had in the past. Also, when patients pay in advance, you'll enjoy another side benefit: They'll find less wrong with your work! When people owe money, they can *claim* that something's wrong with the service or product for which they owe… and thus duck out of their responsibility to pay. Has this ever happened to you?

In short, the key to seeing as few or as many patients as you would like is knowing how to handle the question of payment, so that you can move your patients from an *a la carte* basis to a *prix fixe* approach that benefits them—and you.

8. Have Little or No Accounts Receivables.

There's nothing more frustrating than performing dental work for people who won't pay for it. I've never been in a dental office that didn't have that little plaque that says, "Payment is due at the time services are delivered." I've also never been in a dental office (except for those belonging to my clients, who know better) that didn't have thousands or even tens of thousands of dollars of accounts receivable on the books. If you know how to get your patients to pay in full and to pay in advance, you don't have a lot of accounts receivable.

9. **Delegate all Tasks that You Dislike and Still Retain Complete Control and Accuracy in Your Practice.**

Whenever I come on board with a new client, I'm always shocked to find the degree to which that dentist, like so many dentists who are not achieving their highest level of success, is unable to delegate.

Many dentists suffer a need for compulsive over-control in their workplace. They find it impossible to delegate financial matters to people who are specifically trained to work as bookkeepers or accountants. They meddle in staffing problems that ought to be handled by the office manager or some other designated person. They've constantly got their noses in the appointment book, moving patients around, insisting that people reschedule for the convenience of the dentist and not for the patient. They behave like out-of-control traffic cops, sometimes creating motion and havoc with everybody's schedules for no discernible benefit to anyone. Still other dentists spend valuable time writing up charts instead of having their assistants do that kind of work. They bypass the person accountable for these tasks and, in so doing, invalidate them.

A dentist who does not know how to delegate wastes his or her own time and demeans the entire team. After all, a dentist's team is (at least in theory) trained and competent to complete the tasks that the dentist can't seem to let go of. My clients learn how to delegate all the tasks that they dislike and all the tasks that they shouldn't be involving themselves with, because their time is too valuable.

They end up with an office that runs more smoothly and a team with a much higher level of morale.

10. Work Eighty Percent Chairside, Ten Percent on Managing Your Business, and Ten Percent on Designing Your Future.

As we saw in the previous point, most dentists waste an enormous amount of time managing the wrong things. Not my clients. They spend only ten percent of their time managing the business because they know how to delegate, empower, and avoid undercutting the people they are paying to accomplish things for them. Instead of spending sixty percent of their time chairside, they now spend eighty percent chairside.

In addition to the ten percent of the time managing the business, they spend another ten percent of the time designing the future of the business. This is the sort of advance planning—some might call it dreamwork or just time away or time off—that totally eludes most dentists, who don't have the time for it and don't even know how to go about doing it, even if they could make the time, which is highly unlikely.

11. Have a Team that Motivates You.

Most dentists think that they have the responsibility of motivating their entire team, from the front desk people to the hygienists to the person who books the appointments to the bookkeeper. Most dentists think that they are expected to be a combination of Tony Robbins and Vince Lombardi, imparting motivational thoughts to their teams at all times. The reality is that most dentists are far too frazzled to motivate anybody, including themselves.

I teach my clients that motivation actually flows from the team upward to the dentist, instead of the other way around. I'll show you how to turn every aspect of your practice into a profit center.

You'll discover how to train your dental hygienists to present cases and not just clean teeth, and how to motivate the hygienists, the appointment coordinator, the front desk people, and everyone else in the office. Everyone receives incentives to bring in more revenue for the business. You want to show them how to be entrepreneurial in their outlook and approach to work.

Ironically, the number one complaint I hear from my clients' team members has to do with the fact that the dentists who hired me aren't doing all the dentistry that they took the initiative to sell! Doesn't that sound like the ideal problem to have with your team? That's right—the team is actually pushing the doctor to do more dentistry. Why not you?

12. Have a Team that Respects You and Takes Your Direction.

When the energy of the team is unleashed and team members are encouraged, through direct financial incentives, to be proactive in terms of creating revenue, everybody wins. My clients look at each aspect of their practice—the appointment coordinator, the hygienists, the front desk people—as individuals who are playing a great game, and that game is, "Make more money for the office."

There's no denying that you may be at least in part motivated by money; for most dentists, this is at least one reason why they went into dentistry in the first place. Why should it be any different for your team? When you bring out the entrepreneurial spirit in your team members, they will respect you, appreciate you, and be highly motivated to do whatever it takes to keep their jobs. After all, there exist grapevines among all of the different groups of people who work in dental offices in any city or town. They all know which offices are hot, which offices pay the best, and which offices are the most fun. The people currently working for you will be highly motivated to do the best job possible for you so that they can keep their jobs, because they know that everybody else in town wishes they worked for you. How does that sound? Best of all, you'll no longer be solely responsible for driving your practice. You'll see how everyone else in the office will actually be very excited and motivated to share that all-important responsibility with you.

13. Have a Waiting List of Professionals Demanding to Work for You.

Some dentists have rocky relationships with their team members. Most people—not just dentists—shy away from confrontation, and dentists take the attitude that it's better to have a mediocre team member on board than to have no one at all. Many dentists tell themselves, "There are no good people out there anyway," and they figure the devil they know is better than the devil they don't know.

Other dentists take a very different approach, churning through team members in an effort to find the "perfect" person. This search for perfection inevitably fails, not because the team members are uniformly terrible but because the demands that the dentist places on these people are simply far too high for any reasonable human being, especially for the salaries offered. One of my clients went through seventy-seven people in seven years before he brought me on board. That's no way to run an office.

> ONE OF MY CLIENTS WENT THROUGH SEVENTY-SEVEN PEOPLE IN SEVEN YEARS BEFORE HE BROUGHT ME ON BOARD. THAT'S NO WAY TO RUN AN OFFICE.

The fact is that there are wonderful people out there, and they have enough self-esteem and dignity to work only in wonderful places. If your office transcends the usual sorts of problems by applying the exceptional sorts of solutions that I offer my clients, word will get around the grapevine in your community, and you will be in the delightful position of being able to pick and choose from the best of the best in every aspect of staffing your office.

14. Have Fun and Enjoy Going to the Office Daily.

Most dentists think that they are stuck for life with the stressors that make their lives miserable: recalcitrant team members; nonpaying patients; patients who cancel appointments, show up late, or are simply no-shows. Most dentists think that these aggravating factors are simply part of the cost of doing business. Not my clients, who know how to remove each of these different stressors and thus free themselves from the pain that most dentists experience on a daily basis.

15. Be Recognized by Your Colleagues, Your Team, and Your Community as a Leader in Making a Difference in People's Lives.

It's said that anybody who goes to dental school for the money is not likely to finish dental school. You really have to love people, at least on some level, and you have to be motivated and even inspired to serve. That's true for practically every dentist in the world. The difference is that most dentists are stuck in survival mode, working endless hours so they can keep billing, just to keep their heads above water.

When you can cut your weekly hours down from, say, forty or fifty to twenty-five, that leaves you with plenty of time to serve the community. You can open your office one day a month to residents of a homeless shelter, a shelter for battered women, underprivileged children, or whomsoever you choose. If you are able to select the kind of dental work you would rather practice instead of the drilling, filling, and billing routine that most dentists endure, you will develop a reputation among your peers for that kind of work, and they will be far more likely to refer that kind of work to you. These are only some of the upsides to taking control of your practice and your financial life.

Your colleagues in your community will be well aware of the personality change you'll undergo, if complaining about patients, team, or the practice of dentistry has been a way of life for you. They'll notice your happier demeanor, and they'll sense that something radical has changed for you. And they'll want to know what it is.

16. Maintain Control Over Your Life and Practice No Matter What Breakdowns Come Your Way.

There's no such thing as a breakdown-free existence. Personal problems persist; not all patients are ideal. Life happens. But by taking control of so many aspects of one's life, practice, and finances, the breakdowns that do occur—and they are fewer and further between for my clients—simply don't matter as much. They don't represent the kind of significant setbacks that they might have been in the past. When you're in control of the big things, the little things eliminate themselves—or just don't matter as much anymore.

17. Have a Secure Future; Retire With Peace and Dignity and Leave a Legacy.

Most dentists have no plan for retirement. That's because they can't afford to retire.

They are so deeply imbedded in that financial morass of too many accounts receivable, anemic cash flow, and too many expenses at home that they can't even think about retirement. My clients do have plans for retirement. I ask them whether they want to keep practicing dentistry ten years from now. Together, we work out exactly how many hours—how many highly profitable hours, that is—it would take over a period of how many years in order to retire at whatever age they choose. I show them that it's possible to sell parts of their practice to associates, bank the proceeds, and create investment assets with that money. There are a lot of things dentists would rather do other than practice dentistry all day long, all year long, or throughout their whole lives. I show my clients how to make all their dreams come true.

There you have it—seventeen aspects of the life you are entitled to lead. Freedom from financial pressure, a convivial and focused team, patients who show up for—and pay for—all of the treatment they need: when you put all this together, it adds up to the most elusive benefit of all—*freedom and peace of mind*. Throughout the rest of this book, I'm going to work with you in every aspect of your practice, so that you can make the same transformations my clients have made and you can reap the same benefits they now enjoy.

You've already done the hard work. You survived dental school. You've built a thriving practice. Now it's time to take the next step and get everything out of your education, experience, and hard work that you so richly deserve. In the next chapter, I'll begin to show you how to accomplish just that.

Take Your Practice to the NextLevel:

1. I want you to envision the life you're entitled to lead. It's a life in which your office operates smoothly, your team supports you as never before, your patients show up—on time—and pay for their care in advance, and your stress level radically diminishes. What would you be doing if you weren't stressed or worried about your business? What options would suddenly become available to you?

2. In the life you deserve, you'll no longer have to worry about late, broken, or cancelled appointments, accounts receivable, patients who cause more trouble than they're worth, or team members who disrupt your office. Instead, top professionals will be seeking ways to learn how they can work for you. Take a moment to envision the kind of life you want. Make a list of the things you want to accomplish, both within and beyond your business. Use this as a guidepost to where you want to go.

3. In the life you're meant to have, you'll be recognized as a leader in your field and a contributor to your community. You'll also have the income that will permit you to plan a lifestyle and retirement on your terms.

   Now does that sound like a great life or what? Well, that's the future that you deserve.

Chapter 3

CPR—Cash in Your Pocket Right Now

S O FAR, WE'VE SEEN the kinds of real problems dentists
face in their practices, in their financial lives, and
at home. In Chapter 2, we saw what life can be like for
dentists who take a different approach to the way they run
their offices... and their lives. One of the primary problems
many dentists face has to do with generating enough cash
flow to support the needs of their businesses and their
personal needs as well. So in this chapter, I'd like to share
with you some ideas about what I call financial CPR—Cash
In Your Pocket Right Now.

You can apply some or all of these ideas in your practice
immediately. You'll find additional sums of money flowing
in right away—and the great news is that you don't have to
do any further investing in your business or in hiring a new
staff member to make this income possible.

My philosophy is that dentists succeed not because
of economic conditions but because of the way they view
themselves and their practices. Lots of dentists thrive even

during recessions and downtimes in the economy. The reason they succeed is that they have a willingness to open their minds to new ideas. They are willing to examine and reexamine the beliefs they have about themselves, about what's possible financially in their lives, and about how their offices can run more smoothly. I'd like you to try these ideas on for size yourself. The good news is that they always work—they worked for all of my clients, and they will work for you as well.

Don't expect to find in this chapter "guaranteed" closing scripts, high-pressure sales tactics, or questionable new ways to "persuade." The ideas I'm going to share with you now are honest, straightforward, proven, and extremely powerful. So let's dive right in.

> **DON'T EXPECT TO FIND IN THIS CHAPTER "GUARANTEED" CLOSING SCRIPTS, HIGH-PRESSURE SALES TACTICS, OR QUESTIONABLE NEW WAYS TO "PERSUADE."**

1. Get Paid.

Many dentists have long lists of outstanding balances— patients who have owed them money for weeks, months, or even longer.

It's time to collect.

Appoint a "point person" for handling these debts. Most of the time, offices are scrambling just to keep up with whatever immediate crisis needs attention. Instead, I'd like you to take a different approach. I want you to give that point person—whether it is your office manager or some other individual with good phone skills—dedicated, quiet time so that he or she can focus on this extremely important task. Your point person cannot be on the floor when making these calls. What you really want to do is lock this person up in a room somewhere, and only let him or her come out tens of thousands of dollars later!

Seriously, schedule your point person to come in on his or her off day, or schedule a block of hours for that person when the office isn't expected to be busy. Begin by generating a list of all outstanding balances and the patients who owe them. Then separate that list into two groups: those who are likely to pay if you simply contact them, and those who might be a little more difficult. Have your point person start with the easy ones.

Many dentists fear that if they call patients, asking to be paid, those patients will leave. So you want to start off with your best patients—the ones who understand that they owe money and simply haven't gotten around to sending a check. These people will invariably clean up their debts right on the spot, putting cash in your pocket right now (the theme of this chapter!).

Incidentally, you will lose only the patients you should fire anyway—the ones who have no interest in paying you.

Next, let's deal with the people who use you and your office as a bank. Send them a letter in which you explain that it's just not fair for some patients in your office not to pay for their services. So instead of raising your fees, you've instituted a new policy under which you ask everyone to pay what they owe. You offer different options in order to give the patient an opportunity to correct this situation, which you (meaning your office) have been responsible for permitting to happen.

Here are the financing options you offer: Patients can pay in full right now with a five percent courtesy discount. They can use interest-free third party financing (more about that later in this chapter). Or they can tell your office when they expect to have the entire balance paid in full. Essentially, with that third option, you are making a new agreement, *in writing*, with the patient, because it is likely that the patient never signed off on any sort of verbal or written treatment agreement back when you did the work.

If the money isn't forthcoming, then it's up to you to have your point person follow up with a phone call.

The purpose of this approach is to get agreements from those people who still owe you money, so that you can clean up your past. It's virtually impossible to build a solid financial present or future unless the past is already handled. Most dentists think that they constantly need a higher and higher number of new patients. The reality is that they just have to go back and collect what is owed to them, and then they won't need to churn quite so many people through the office.

If you get paid on your past due accounts and get paid on time with the new work you do, you'll enjoy an abundance of cash rolling into your office.

Again, the only thing that keeps most dentists from seeking payment for work from their late-paying patients is the fear that those patients will leave. Think about it this way: You are extending no-interest loans to patients you should have no interest in keeping!

Another way to understand this is to think of it in terms of the difference between scarcity thinking and abundance thinking. Most people think in terms of scarcity—they fear that there isn't enough, and if they don't scramble, they won't get what they need in life. I want you to take a different point of view—I want you to begin to accept the idea that we live in an abundant universe. Without sounding too woo-woo, there really is enough to go around, especially in our society, and especially for people who have the right to practice dentistry! There's no benefit to hanging onto patients who aren't going to pay. It's frustrating, it's upsetting to you, and it does nothing for your bottom line.

THE ONLY THING THAT KEEPS MOST DENTISTS FROM SEEKING PAYMENT FOR WORK FROM THEIR LATE-PAYING PATIENTS IS THE FEAR THAT THOSE PATIENTS WILL LEAVE.

So have your point person first contact the people who will pay, and then contact the people who might pay, and thus you can put money in your pocket right now for work you have already performed—without doing an additional minute of dentistry and without finding an additional new patient.

2. Bring Accountability to the Front Desk.

On a baseball team, everybody has a specific role to play. The pitcher pitches, the shortstop plays short, and they don't suddenly switch positions in the middle of the game. Your front desk ought to be the same way.

In most dentists' offices, the front desk has no account-ability whatsoever. Oh, they all have jobs to do—they mind the appointment book, locate charts that have somehow fallen between the file cabinets, call patients to remind them of upcoming appointments, make coffee. But the reality is that when everyone is responsible for everything, no one is truly responsible for anything.

> **THE REALITY IS THAT WHEN EVERYONE IS RESPONSIBLE FOR EVERYTHING, NO ONE IS TRULY RESPONSIBLE FOR ANYTHING.**

I want you to begin to move your front desk people into two specific positions: an appointment coordinator, to manage your time, and a treatment coordinator, to manage your finances. Ultimately, you want these individuals to be spending eighty percent of their time on those tasks. Otherwise, they will simply do the easiest, least confron-tational things in the world, like confirming appointments. Meanwhile, if they don't fill the appointment book prop-erly, your precious time is lost forever. And if they don't coordinate treatment with good agreements, you'll be back to where you were, with lots of accounts receivable.

Also, you don't want to have to be working on a patient while worrying whether Annie is on the phone at the front desk finding someone to come in and fill the suddenly vacant four o'clock. You want to keep your energies focused on practicing dentistry, not on making sure that other people are doing what they're supposed to do.

What exactly are these new positions, appointment coordinator and treatment coordinator?

The appointment coordinator has the responsibility of maximizing the effectiveness of your time. You want to set up a game with your appointment coordinator. Let's say you are a two-doctor, two-hygienist office. Let's say you'd like to have the office gross $2 million a year, while you only work sixteen days a month. Sound good so far?

Two million dollars a year breaks down to roughly $166,000 a month. If you want to work only sixteen days, your office has to generate $10,000 a day for each of those sixteen days. This means that each doctor should do $4,000 worth of dentistry a day and each of your hygienists should do $1,000 worth of work as well. Two doctors each grossing $4,000, plus two hygienists each grossing $1,000, equals that $10,000 a day. Multiply that $10,000 a day by the sixteen days you want to work (incidentally, that's just four days a week, with no nights or weekends). That's $160,000 a month… and that's just shy of two million a year.

Compensate your appointment coordinator based on her ability to reach that financial goal. Give her a bonus of $10 per provider per day that she books $4,000 worth of dentistry for each of the doctors and $1,000 worth of services for each hygienist. Many dentists worry about how much they'll have to shell out in bonuses, so let's take a look. Your maximum exposure equals four providers a day times ten dollars a day times sixteen working days a month. That's a maximum possible $640 a month, in exchange for which you'll be hitting your goal of approximately $2 million. Not a bad return on investment, wouldn't you agree?

Let's take a deeper look at the numbers. You'll find that your dedicated appointment coordinator will pay for herself from day one. If you pay her $12 an hour for eight hours, that works out, taxes included, to around $100 a day. A typical dentist, prior to the implementation of this system, often makes $400 or more per hour. If the appointment coordinator fills and keeps just one additional hour that would have gone open had she not been serving as your dedicated appointment coordinator, *you made money.* And that's just if she filled in that one extra hour. Imagine if you were compensating her with bonuses on a daily basis, so that she makes those goals every day.

To return to our baseball metaphor, fans and players alike sometimes forget that April games count as much as September games in the standings. It all adds up. In your office, you want to act as if every day was the World Series of cash flow. Most dental offices pay bonuses based on what their people do every month or even every year. These bonuses are often tied to a metric or statistic that has nothing to do with the actual job descriptions of the team members. For example, an assistant may receive a bonus for collections, an aspect of the practice with which she has no actual connection.

That method doesn't work, because people only start to focus on what they are earning or what they should be doing once bonus time rolls around. Or they're helpless to affect their bonuses, because there's no connection between what they do and what they can earn bonuses for. Sure, it's great to have a team that plays their September games with intensity. But you want them just as focused on those April dates as well! How do you make this happen? Have bonuses accrue on a daily and hourly basis. I'll show you how to do this later on, but this is the approach you want to begin to take.

You also want to turn one of your people into a treatment coordinator. This is an individual who closes cases, especially when your patients come out of hygiene. Here's how it works—the patient has his teeth cleaned with the hygienist, who notices and points out specific dental work that is necessary (and accrues a bonus for all cases that she initiates). In most offices, the patient goes directly from the hygienist to the front desk, to schedule an appointment. But the patient has not really agreed to any treatment. In fact, the patient may be simply making an appointment just to save face—he or she may have no intention of following through and actually showing up for the work.

That's not acceptable anymore.

In your new approach to practicing dentistry, make sure that your hygienist turns the patient over not to the front desk, but to your dedicated treatment coordinator. Your treatment coordinator will close the deal, get an agreement from the patient to show up, and have the patient agree to *pay in advance*, or at the latest, when the case is completed.

Once people have made *written* agreements as to the treatment to be delivered and the terms of payment, they rarely back out of them. This is doubly true if they have put their money where their mouth is! (Couldn't resist that one!)

Incidentally, your treatment coordinator is also the person who will explain to new patients that "we are a zero balance office." You want to have that phrase tattooed on everybody's minds! A "zero balance office" is an office where patients are expected to pay in advance or when the case is completed. That way, you have no more accounts receivable—you just have cash in the bank.

> **A "ZERO BALANCE OFFICE" IS AN OFFICE WHERE PATIENTS ARE EXPECTED TO PAY IN ADVANCE OR WHEN THE CASE IS COMPLETED.**

3. Establish an Agreement Among all Team Members as to the Standard for a Completely Healthy Mouth.

Typically, I'll go into an office and meet with the dentists and hygienists and ask this question: "On a scale of 1 to 100, how many of the patients you treat have a completely healthy mouth?" The dentists will routinely say about thirty percent of the patients.

The hygienists will roll their eyes. Their typical answer: one percent.

Most dentists' offices have no standard at all, let alone a common standard, for what constitutes a Completely Healthy Mouth. Once you establish this criterion, you will find that eighty to ninety percent of *all* existing patients need some form of treatment. What's a Completely Healthy Mouth? One in which all soft tissue is completely healthy, with no bleeding points and no recession. Moreover, there is no decay in the hard tissue. This should be your standard, and nothing less.

For example, at what point does your office put in a crown versus putting in fillings? There has to be a uniformly agreed-upon standard, and it may well take your office days of discussion to determine exactly what that dividing line is. Get agreement among all practitioners in your office as to the precise dividing line, so that you are all practicing dentistry in a uniform manner.

If you establish such standards throughout your office, you will soon find that you have so much work to do on your existing patients that you'll need very few new ones (as we'll discuss in greater detail in Chapters 8 and 9).

Once you can recommend necessary treatment to existing patients, your monthly production will skyrocket. It's easier to sell cases to existing patients because you already have a relationship with them. This way, you don't have to worry so much about where the new patients are going to come from. Instead of focusing, as do most dentists (and most businesses) on finding new patients (or customers), you can most likely do a much better job serving the people who already come to you. You're in the business of providing dentistry so that people have healthy mouths.

You're not in the business of "watching" their soft and hard tissue decay. Don't be afraid to do your job to the fullest. From now on, you stand for making sure that every patient enjoys the benefits of having a Completely Healthy Mouth.

Under no circumstances am I advocating that a dentist sell a case for which there is no need. The simple fact is that most people are in such great need of dental care that if you make the "healthy mouth" I described above as your standard—and the uniform standard throughout your office, to which everyone on your team signs on—you will not need another new patient for a long, long time.

4. **Dust Off Your Intraoral Camera and Have Your Hygienist Have at Least Four Shots of Problem Areas Up When You Enter the Hygiene Room for a Re-care Visit.**

Chances are that you already have an intraoral camera, which offers a ten-times-actual-size blowup of situations in a patient's mouth. On the intraoral camera, a filling looks like the Grand Canyon, and as for gum recession… there aren't any words. Most dentists have intraoral cameras, yet few of them use these expensive devices. If you don't show the patient what's wrong, how could the patient possibly understand the nature of the problem? That's actually the job of the hygienist, so that by the time the dentist comes into the room, all the dentist has to do is go over the necessary treatment instead of wasting valuable time convincing the patient that there really is a problem.

Remember that most people don't think they have anything wrong with their mouths. That's a simple fact of the dental profession—people figure that as long as nothing is hurting or falling out, everything is fine. They have been trained—by dentists!—to harbor that notion, simply because dentists have been telling their patients for decades that "we'll just watch that." Patients assume that if something bears watching, it doesn't need action.

You have to interrupt that mindset, and it's really not that hard. Have your hygienist show the patient the problem with at least four shots of problem areas. The patient will understand that work is necessary. And then when you come into the hygienist's room, the patient will be listening very carefully to what you have to say about how to rectify what is clearly an unacceptable situation. If you do not establish a patient's condition as unacceptable—and gain his or her agreement that the situation is unacceptable—stop. Do not present the solution; you'll just be wasting your time.

I started this chapter by saying that you don't have to spend any money to increase your income by following the guidance in this chapter. That point holds true here as well. If you don't have an intraoral camera, don't buy one right now. Many dentists think that if they just keep buying new gear, they can spend their way out of their financial problems. Obviously, you can see the fallacious nature of that thinking. If you don't have an intraoral camera, just ask the hygienist to have the mirror in place, so the patient can see what's wrong. We'll go more deeply into this process in the next chapter. The main point is that you want your hygienist to show the patient exactly what's wrong before you ever step into the hygienist's room to discuss treatment.

5. When Presenting to the Patient, Always Describe First the Problem, then the Consequences if Left Untreated, and Only after that the Solution.

Dentists, who may be driven by fear of inadequate cash flow, tend to go right to the solution. "Mr. Smith, you need two fillings and one crown." Again, the patient is sitting there thinking, "It doesn't hurt, and I've been okay up until now. I don't need this." You won't make a case that way, and if the patient doesn't show up for the treatment that you have prescribed in this manner, don't be surprised.

You may be practicing dentistry, but you are also engaged in a business dependent on sales. If you and the people around you don't sell, you can't work. So you want to keep in mind the basic ideas about selling that govern all businesses. Specifically, consumers buy for one or both of two reasons—either to solve a problem or to make themselves feel good about the purchase they made. You buy things because you want to feel good about yourself. Most people don't feel good about getting dental work done, unless it's cosmetic dentistry. So your job is to show that you are providing a solution to a problem. A solution offered in the abstract will not lead to the patient accepting the case.

Let's review an important point we made earlier. Once you have presented, don't let the patient go off to the front desk to schedule an appointment. Keep in mind that a patient is not likely to confront you and say no. A patient sitting in a dental chair is in a vulnerable position. You have to get that patient to agree to the treatment—and the way you do that is by handing the patient off not to the front desk but to your treatment coordinator. The treatment coordinator will make the agreement with the patient we discussed earlier—the type of treatment, the fee, the treatment schedule, and *the manner in which the fee will be paid.* The treatment coordinator will also handle any questions the patient may have with regard to the treatment. You want your patient to go home with a clear plan for treatment and payment, not worries, questions, or doubts. This is the key element in virtually eliminating broken and cancelled appointments. Failure to do so means that the patient will exaggerate in his or her mind the pain in the mouth and the wallet or purse, and will be far less likely to show up for treatment.

6. Keep Track of Important Statistics Every Day.

Most dentists have absolutely no idea of how much treatment they present in a given day and how much treatment is accepted, both for their new patients and their existing patients. They have no idea of how much production they are doing and how collections are going. They have no concept of the number of new patients coming into their office each month. And they have zero idea of how many broken or cancelled appointments there are in a day. Deputize someone in your office to maintain accurate statistics about all of this information, especially with regard to the vital question of how much treatment you are presenting and how much treatment is accepted, both by new and existing patients. What can be measured can be improved. Tracking these numbers gets your office off the cash-flow roller coaster and will help you predict your future production and cash flow.

7. Slow Down!

A busy schedule is not always a productive schedule. Most dentists feel that if their offices aren't running at a frenetic pace, nothing good is happening. Or they might wish that they could practice dentistry in a more relaxed fashion, but they know they can't, simply because they have to "drill, fill, and bill" just to keep up with their cash flow obligations. That's why I end up suggesting to many of my clients that they have to slow down, take a deep breath, and ask themselves whether all that frenetic activity really is healthy for their bottom line—or for their own well-being and longevity.

It's better to see fewer patients who match your practice philosophy than to try to be all things to all people. A career in dentistry is not a hundred-yard dash. It's a marathon, and pacing is essential.

8. Come Face to Face with the Person or Thing You have been Avoiding, and Take Action Immediately.

We'll talk about this in greater detail in Chapter 5. For now, though, let's discuss a key way to eliminate a serious cause of distraction in your office. This distraction is intangible and often hard to quantify, but it actually costs an office hundreds of thousands of dollars a year if left unchecked.

Many offices have team members who behave in a most unprofessional manner. That person might show up late on a regular basis, come in hung over, call in sick and appear the next day with a nice tan, or cause upsets with other team members. Today—right now—go over to that person and bring that person into your office, and name the game: tell the person exactly what he or she is doing, and explain that that behavior does not match your expectations for professionalism.

Don't know what to say? Try this: "It's no longer acceptable that you operate this way." Leave the meeting with an agreement from that person as to how things will go in the future. And if the person continues to behave in that unacceptable manner, follow up with a verbal warning, a written warning, and finally dismissal.

Most dentists simply do not realize the amount of time, money, and energy that they spend by keeping on their teams those individuals who simply do not know how to behave in an appropriate manner.

Basically, there are three types of team members—those who are open and willing, those who are negative, and those who are outright thieves. You can work only with the willing. You've got to face any employee who is distracting you and your practice from reaching your goals. I tell my clients to hire slowly and fire fast. Take your time so that you get a really quality person on board, instead of doing what too many dentists do: simply hiring the next pretty face or even the next person with a pulse who comes along. And above all, don't keep troublesome people on your payroll. Confront them and give them an opportunity to correct themselves. If they do not, then relieve them of their duties.

9. Fire Problem Patients.

Have the courage to fire your problem patients. They probably don't even pay you, and even if they do, you could easily
replace that income many times over with the amount of
mental energy they consume—and the anguish they cause.
Let them find some other dentist to annoy.

10. Pay Your Own Bills on Time… and Show Up on Time for Your Own Commitments.

When you pay your own bills on time, people pay you on
time. I call it the Zen form of accounts receivable. After all,
if you have outstanding balances with your vendors, you
have no right to expect other people to pay you on time. I'd
like to share a simple solution with you. Countless credit
card companies are falling over each other trying to extend
interest-free loans to high-income and high-status individuals like you. Take advantage of one of these offers—borrow
money from a credit card company at zero percent interest for six months. Pay off all your outstanding debts and
your credit card balances. Six months from now, when the
bill comes due for this loan, you'll have more than enough
money to pay it off instantly because of this cash-generat-
ing system you're installing at work.

Now let's talk about time. What applies to money applies
to time as well. If you show up late and constantly rearrange
your schedule and the schedules of everyone around you,
your patients and team will believe that this is acceptable

conduct. Start on time, and see people on time. Correcting this time issue will transform the way your patients relate to you. Your team's accountability rises and falls with your own.

I charge my dentist clients $100 a minute for every minute they are late to our appointments. I don't tolerate lateness, in myself or in others, and neither should you. Yes, certainly there are moments when lateness is unavoidable. But I'm talking about those who run late consistently. That behavior is simply unacceptable.

The wife of one of my clients once approached me and said, "I know my husband is responsible at work, but I can't count on him at home. Can you do anything about that for me?"

I called up the dentist and said, "Do you want to play a game?"

"Sure, what is it?"

"I want you to pay your wife a thousand dollars for every broken agreement."

He agreed. That day, his wife asked him to clean the garage. He said he would, but he didn't get around to it for a week. He ended up writing her a check for $7,000!

At his twentieth college reunion, which followed shortly after this experience, he and all the rest of his classmates were asked what was the most important thing they had learned in their twenty years since graduation. He told his classmates, "Clean your garage!" What he meant was that it is vital to keep your word at the office… and at home.

11. Cancel Your Yellow Pages Ad.

It's a tradition for a dentist to run an ad in the Yellow Pages. But so what? Yellow Pages ads very rarely return their full investment, unless you specialize in sedation dentistry. Patients do not make a buying decision to do cosmetic dentistry or other expensive forms of dentistry because of ads in the Yellow Pages. On top of that, there are two major competing books, and then you've also got the Internet. These factors diminish the usefulness of Yellow Pages ads, and you end up getting the wrong type of patient.

The people who come to you shouldn't come from the Yellow Pages. They should come from referrals—satisfied, happy patients who appreciate the professionalism of you and your office, who pay in advance or when the case is inserted, and who have friends who live their lives in exactly the same manner. Let your fingers do the walking… somewhere else.

12. Offer Three Payment Options.

Again, stop being the bank. As I mentioned, my clients allow their patients to pay in full at the time of treatment with one "bookkeeping courtesy" of five percent. I've found that ninety- nine percent of dental offices have tried CareCredit or Dental Fee Plan, but most dentists' offices simply don't know how to use these plans. CareCredit and DFP constitute hugely powerful closing tools, but only if you and your team know how to use them properly. Yes, there is a fee for using these plans, but there's a much higher cost to having outstanding receivables. Essentially, you want to sell the dentistry, and at the same time, you want to show the patient how to pay. More about this in a later chapter. The third option: one-half payment upon agreement and one-half on a specifically agreed-upon date before the case is completed. Make a new agreement… and then hold your patient to that agreement.

13. Quit Tearing Up Hundreds of "Four-Dollar Bills" Every Month.

What's a four-dollar bill? Every bill you send from your office costs you an average of four bucks. Most offices send out two hundred to three hundred bills a month, a shockingly high percentage of which are routinely ignored by their patients. This triggers the need to send out another bill, and another bill, and another bill, until you give up or retire from dentistry. Get off the mailing merry-go-round by having a dedicated team person making calls to patients, who will either give credit card numbers over the phone or commit to sending in a check, as we discussed in item one of this chapter. That way, you can take the eight hundred to twelve hundred dollars a month that you've been spending on bills that go nowhere and put that money where it belongs—on the lease payment for your new 7 Series.

14. Present Comprehensive, Preventative Care to Each and Every Patient.

You cannot be afraid to present comprehensive, preventative care to each patient. You are your patient's sole trusted advisor when it comes to their dental health. They're counting on you to tell them what is necessary, so don't let them down by failing to present cases simply because you are afraid of rejection or for any other reason. This is a vital point, and we will come back to it a number of different times in this book.

> **YOU CANNOT BE AFRAID TO PRESENT COMPREHENSIVE, PREVENTATIVE CARE TO EACH PATIENT. YOU ARE YOUR PATIENT'S SOLE TRUSTED ADVISOR WHEN IT COMES TO THEIR DENTAL HEALTH.**

15. Pay Off All High-Interest Debt, Including Credit Cards.

Dentists often get in arrears with suppliers because they—and their spouses—believe they deserve to lead a certain kind of upscale lifestyle. These dentists "rob" their businesses by taking more in salary than the practice actually collects. Many things contribute to this accounts receivable crisis. Do you really need to carry all that credit card debt? Pay it down, and pay cash from now on. Use the new money you're making as a result of the ideas in this chapter to pay off your credit cards, once and for all.

16. Finally, Do Not Try to Be Everything to All People.

I want to introduce you to a concept called the QSP Positioning Guide. The three aspects of the QSP Positioning

Guide are quality, service, and price. A good business can offer two of the three, but not all three. Let's see how this works.

If you want quality and service when you stay at a hotel, you'll go to a Ritz-Carlton. If you want quality and service when you buy jewelry, you'll visit Tiffany's. In neither case will you expect to find the vendor competitive in terms of price. These businesses focus on quality and service for a clientele that is not scared off by relatively high prices.

If you want quality and price, you can go to a Costco or a WalMart, but you might get run over by a forklift in one of those huge warehouse stores. Or if you want a lawnmower, you'll have to buy six of them that are shrink-wrapped together. The quality and prices cannot be beat in stores like this, but if you're looking for service, you may be looking a long time.

Finally, you've got businesses like McDonald's, which provide great service. You're in and out in seven minutes or less. They also provide low prices, like the Dollar Menu. But is the quality there?

Of these three businesses, which one is right? The simple answer is that they're all right. Each of these businesses focuses on two aspects of the QSP Positioning Guide and ignores the third. But what about you?

Most dentists run into trouble because they try to serve everyone. The idea of QSP simply hasn't been on their radar. You want to eliminate confusion. You're most likely going to be about quality and service, and that means that you don't have to compromise on price. I tell my clients to tell their patients, "We offer high quality and impeccable service, and it costs money to offer this. If you don't want that, if you don't care about the best quality of materials, there are plenty of places to go for a lower level of treatment."

Again, it comes back to that earlier idea we mentioned regarding scarcity and abundance. If a dentist embraces a point of view based on scarcity, that dentist will scrap for every possible client and will never turn down any work. As a result, that dentist will have a muddled image in the community. But if a dentist believes in the abundance of the kind of patients he or she really wants to treat, that dentist will find those patients—and will thrive treating them. None of us can be all things to all people. Choose your two sides of the QSP Positioning Guide, and act accordingly.

These sixteen ideas are guaranteed to perform CPR on your dental practice—to put Cash In Your Pocket Right Now. In succeeding chapters, I'd like to take you deeper into each of the ideas we discussed in this chapter and show you exactly what my clients do, so that they can practice as much or as little dentistry as they choose, have their offices running more smoothly than they could ever believe, and make far more money—in far less time, with far less stress—than they ever thought imaginable. We'll begin with the age-old question of what you really should be doing with your dental hygienist in the next chapter.

Take Your Practice to the NextLevel:

1. You can put "cash in your pocket right now" simply by collecting the fees you are currently owed.

    a. Enroll someone in your office to make calls and collect fees. Create a game to pay this person per call, per collection, or by a percentage.

    b. Invest in good training for your collections person. Make it a point to support your collections person, reminding him or her to not take it personally if people are rude. Create games that make the rejection acceptable and even fun.

2. Create the positions of appointment coordinator and treatment coordinator, and give these employees bonuses that track their performance on an hour-by-hour and day-by-day basis.

3. Make your office a "zero balance office" to eliminate accounts receivable, which amount to interest-free loans for your patients. For more info on how to be effective using third party financing, download CCWare at CareCredit.com.

4. Problem patients—and problematic team members—have no place in your office. You are only as strong as your weakest link.

Chapter 4

What You Really Should be Doing with Your Dental Hygienist

I F YOU'RE LIKE MOST dentists, you turned to this chapter first!

The real purpose of this chapter is to give you some ideas about how to make your dental hygienist the catalyst of a perpetual motion dental practice money machine. The ideas I am going to share with you generate a huge amount of cash for my clients.

Most dentists tend to look at their hygienists as a cost to the practice. They say, "I'm paying my hygienist good money, and I just want my money's worth." As a result, some dentists will insist that the hygienist actually squeeze in two patients an hour, instead of giving each patient all the time that he or she really needs. Worst of all, most dentists fail to recognize that they can build a substantial dental practice if only they would utilize their hygienists to do the following:

- Recognize problems.

- Educate patients about the nature of those problems.

- Point out those problems to the dentist when he or she comes into hygiene to visit with a patient.

Simply put, the hygienists my clients employ now generate $30,000 to $50,000 a month in new cases, which means as much as *half a million dollars or more per hygienist* in additional income generated for their dentists each year. If your hygienist isn't generating that kind of income for you, then you are leaving an awful lot of money on the table.

I want to show you how to turn your hygienist into a profit center and how to make her the cornerstone of the dental care delivery system in your office. But before we get into the specifics of how to do that, let's review the three ways to build a practice.

I WANT TO SHOW YOU HOW TO TURN YOUR HYGIENIST INTO A PROFIT CENTER AND HOW TO MAKE HER THE CORNERSTONE OF THE DENTAL CARE DELIVERY SYSTEM IN YOUR OFFICE.

The hardest way to build a practice—and most frequently the first choice of dentists—is through bringing in new patients. The problem is that it's hard work and expensive—to create a constant flow of new patients. This is simply the toughest way to build a dental practice, because it relies on a churn-and-burn philosophy. You're not getting off the treadmill by increasing the number of new patients you see. You're simply causing the treadmill to run faster and faster. That's detrimental to your health, to the peace and serenity of your office, and to your bottom line.

The second way to build a dental practice is to have your existing patients increase the frequency of their visits. This is easier than trying to generate a constant stream of new faces, and it requires your office to be considerably more efficient in implementing its re-care system. The problem is that most dentists allow patients to fall out of the system, to slip through the cracks, and to fail to reappear for regular re-care visits. The other problem is that most dentists rely on hope and prayer to close cases. Unless you've got a better way of closing cases, you're not going to increase your business in any meaningful way simply by getting your existing patients to return more frequently.

It doesn't really help to have patients coming through your office if you keep telling them the same thing over and over again—"We're going to watch that," "Let's see what happens with that in a few months," and all the other clichés that dentists use. Why do dentists resort to these clichés? Most of the time, it's in order to avoid the rejection they may face when they present cases to their patients.

In short, bringing your existing patients back more frequently for re-care visits is a step up from trying to find new ways to bring in a constant flow of fresh new patients, but the benefit to your bottom line is marginal.

The easiest way to build your dental practice in a significant manner is to get your existing patients to accept at least eighty percent of the treatment presented. You've already got people coming through your office whose mouths don't match the "healthy mouth" standard we discussed in the previous chapter—healthy soft tissue and healthy hard tissue. If you could sell them on the services they truly need eighty percent of the time—and I can show you how to do that—you wouldn't need to keep churning new patients.

In my consulting work with dentists, I have come to the surprising discovery that in the average dental office, new patients accept only seventeen percent of the treatment proposed to them. Or to put it another way, eighty-three percent of the treatment that dentists propose is rejected. No wonder dentists become gun shy about presenting comprehensive care.

The numbers are better for existing patients, but they're nothing to get excited about. The average dental practice only closes thirty-four percent of the treatment proposed. My clients raise their rate of closing cases for new patients to sixty percent, and they close cases with their existing patients over eighty percent of the time. They do this by making efficient use of their hygiene program. To put it simply, patient education—and therefore the closing of cases—starts in hygiene.

Just as your dental hygienist does not want to work the phones, your dental hygienist also does not want to go into sales. Hygienists don't like the term "sales." They do love the term "patient education," and they do love getting paid. So from now on, you want to have your hygienist educate patients about problems in their mouths and the consequences that will follow if those problems are not treated. Your hygienist shouldn't come out and say definitely, "You'll need a crown for that tooth." Instead, your hygienist should suggest that you are likely to propose a crown, given the situation that she sees. She is foreshadowing the solutions that you'll offer when you step into her room to see the patient. But by the time you come in, the hygienist should have educated the patient thoroughly about the nature of the problems that he or she is presenting and the consequences if those problems are left untreated.

How do you motivate a hygienist to provide this level of patient education? First, don't give her just half an hour or forty-five minutes per patient. *Give her a full hour.* Over the course of that hour, she will have all the time she needs in order to do her hygiene work at the highest level, and then she will have all the time she needs in order to provide the patient education that you want—and need her to provide. Second, *pay your dental hygienist one percent of everything your office makes* on cases that originate from the patient education she provides. This one percent is over and above the amount that you are paying her in salary.

Again, dental hygienists do not want to work the phones, they do not want to be telemarketers, and they do not want to go into sales. They went to hygiene school in order to learn how to do preventative care on teeth and gums and to help people maintain healthy mouths. So allow your dental hygienist to achieve her main purpose in life. At the same time, share with her the fact that you want her to provide a much higher level of patient education than in the past, and that you will compensate her for work that is generated in this manner.

You want your hygienist to be very clear with you, with herself, and with your patients about the precise nature of her purpose. I counsel my clients to have their hygienists write up their own personal statements of purpose and post those statements in their rooms. One example: "My commitment to my patients—to help you achieve and maintain completely healthy teeth and gums, for the rest of your life."

Tell your hygienist that you are not expecting her to sell. However, you may want to mention to her that there's nothing to be ashamed of with regard to the selling process. After all, if patients aren't informed of and sold on the care they need, they won't have healthy mouths, and that ultimately defeats her purpose as a dental hygienist and your purpose as a dentist. You might even want to tell her that the root of the word "sales" is "assisting," not persuading or making people do something they don't want to do. The main thing is that you want to stress with her that she is *providing patient education*—she is *not* selling.

> **AFTER ALL, IF PATIENTS AREN'T INFORMED OF AND SOLD ON THE CARE THEY NEED, THEY WON'T HAVE HEALTHY MOUTHS, AND THAT ULTIMATELY DEFEATS HER PURPOSE AS A DENTAL HYGIENIST AND YOUR PURPOSE AS A DENTIST.**

What does a practice look like when the hygienist is committed to this level of patient education and has the time in order to do her job—and provide this new higher level of patient education—properly?

First, she isn't diagnosing. She is simply pointing out problems. To that end, neither she nor you should be performing "wallet biopsies" on patients. So often, dentists and hygienists only present cases to the limit of what they think the patient can pay for or their insurance can pay for. Tell your hygienist not to worry about how the patient is going to pay for the service. If the patient asks the hygienist, "Is it going to cost a lot?" then train your hygienist to offer this answer: "I understand your concern about your investment in your care. After we're finished, I'm going to take you to the treatment coordinator. We have different types of payment options to meet your budget, and the treatment coordinator will help you with the budgeting, so it will all work for you."

A script like this will give your dental hygienist confidence when people raise that question about money. The specific wording I am suggesting will assuage your patient's fears about how he or she is going to handle this new financial burden. Your dental hygienist thus can focus specifically on the thing that makes her happiest—taking care of her patients' dental hygiene needs and demonstrating to the patient the problems and the consequences of those problems if left untreated. These are the tasks she feels motivated to perform. And then when you pay her one percent of all the cases that close and are completed, she becomes deeply invested in making sure that neither you nor anyone else in the office drops the ball on getting that work done.

Second, this approach maximizes the use of your precious time. By the time you walk into hygiene to meet the patient, your hygienist has already put up four pictures of the problem on the intraoral camera or has positioned the mirror so that the problems are visible to the patient. By now, incidentally, you've solved your immediate cash-flow problem, thanks to the solutions we discussed in the previous chapter. I now want to recommend the best possible investment for your practice: the intraoral camera. If you know how to use it, it will repay its own cost within a single week. If you do not have an intraoral camera, go get one—as soon as you can. It is the single most important and lucrative tool your office could possibly have when it comes to presenting and closing cases. When the patient sees four views of the problem or problems magnified on the screen, your patient is going to be far more likely to accept the case.

The key element in shifting from selling the patient to having the patient buy is transferring your attention on what you want to having the patient see the problem. Self-discovery by patients enrolls them in their treatment. This is what I call "the moment of truth," when the patient tells you, "Doctor, let's take care of this problem."

When your hygienist, motivated by her desire to care for your patients' teeth and mouths, and also motivated by that additional one percent she's going to make, has performed her patient education role, then and only then do you come in to hygiene. Instead of spending a long, laborious time with the patient, where you are essentially starting from scratch, trying to figure out what, if anything, the dental hygienist has accomplished in terms of patient education, now the hygienist is expecting you to come in to confirm the case that she has already presented. This is only going to take you five minutes.

You don't have to do a whole lot of selling—the views presented on the intraoral camera will speak volumes. If the patient asks you about the cost of the care, tell the patient the same thing the hygienist said—the treatment coordinator will discuss payment options with you. You spend an efficient five minutes with the patient, and then you're out of there, off to do something else that makes an equally efficient use of your time.

Why all this emphasis on patient education? Let me ask you this question. When was the last time you made a buying decision that cost you $5,000 to $8,000 when you didn't even *know* you had a problem, when you were in a vulnerable position like a dental chair, when you didn't want to make that purchase, and when you weren't feeling any pain or discomfort that made you think you needed that purchase in the first place? Keep in mind that for years now, you've been probably telling your patients, "We'll put a watch on that." In other words, most dentists have conditioned their patients to believe that unless something is hurting or falling out of their mouths, they don't need any treatment!

That's why patient education is so important, and *it's not your job*. It *is* the job of the dental hygienist, because she can tell the patient what the problem is and what the consequences are, in a non-threatening way.

Third, by coming in and seeing what she's put up on the

intraoral camera, the dentist is far less likely to undercut the hygienist—something that happens accidentally, but all too often. Here's how the situation usually unfolds. First, the dental hygienist will present problems to the patient, and the patient is in accord with the idea that something needs to be done. And then the dentist enters, concerned that if he presents an expensive case he might be rejected. That fear of rejection may actually cause him to invalidate everything the hygienist so accurately pointed out to the patient.

The dentist, afraid of rejection, says things like, "We're not going to do that" or "We're going to watch that" or "We'll take it easy on that." This results in the hygienist becoming gun-shy about presenting. You've got to trust the fact that your hygienist knows what's going on inside a mouth. So instead of invalidating her, accustom yourself to acknowledge her for what she found. Tell her, *in front of the patient*, "It's great that you found that!" Find her doing things the right way, and acknowledge her for it.

When your hygienist is performing her role, she is likely to generate that $30,000 to $50,000 a month in additional work for you. Here's how it happens: You've got a dedicated appointment coordinator, who is making sure that every one of your hygienist's slots is full. She's got an hour for each patient, more than enough time for her to provide the care she needs and offer the education that you want her to provide. She then suggests the care that is needed or at least presents the problems and potential consequences. You enter and spend five minutes confirming the findings. The hygienist then brings the patient not to the front desk or to the front door, but instead to the treatment coordinator, who essentially closes the deal. And then, when that case closes, is completed, *and is paid for*, your hygienist gets one percent of the deal.

WHEN YOUR HYGIENIST IS PERFORMING HER ROLE, SHE IS LIKELY TO GENERATE THAT $30,000 TO $50,000 A MONTH IN ADDITIONAL WORK FOR YOU.

After each patient has come through hygiene, the hygienist needs to fill out a Hygiene Tracking Form, which should include the name of the patient, the actual treatment presented, and the treatment accepted. Your hygienist has access to those forms at all times. This way, she can keep track of how much of the case has closed. In fact, she is going to be bugging your treatment coordinator to make sure that the case is closed. That's the way it should be—you want everybody in your office to be focused on making sure that all cases close, get done, and get paid for in full.

Just as the dental hygienist gets one percent for all work that is completed and then paid for, the treatment coordinator also gets one percent. This will guarantee that the treatment coordinator is just as concerned as the hygienist that you don't drop the ball and that you complete—and make sure that you get paid for—all this extra work.

You might say, "I don't want to pay these people all that much money." In reality, the bigger the checks you write to your dental hygienist and your treatment coordinator, based on those one percent bonuses, the happier you should be—because the other ninety-eight percent (after those two bonuses of one percent each) is money that flows to your bottom line only because this system is in effect. *The additional income that you're earning as a result of this system is practically pure profit, because the only expenses associated with this income relate to the bonuses, lab work, and supplies. On average, about eighty percent of the income you'll generate this way goes directly to your bottom line.*

Take it a step further. Have your hygienist introduce other products such as Invisalign and whitening. Think of the benefits to your patients, who would love to have these products explained to them. And think of the benefit to the bottom line in your office.

Products like Invisalign and whitening will never be mentioned unless you and your hygienist have this system in place, by which you are tracking and rewarding her for all the work that she generates.

Let's say you're with me so far—the hygienist now gets an hour to do her thing, you come in for five minutes to confirm problems she identified, and the treatment coordinator closes the deal, arranges payment, and makes additional appointments, if necessary. When you employ this system, you'll want to make sure that your hygienist has a patient in her chair every hour she's at work. Why? Because every patient she educates is likely to produce additional, high-profit income for you. Every hour she's not working is costing you a lot of money. So how do you ensure that your hygienist is always with a patient?

The solution: Hire a new part-time individual in your office—a re-care coordinator. The role of the re-care coordinator is to make sure that there is someone in your hygienist's chair every single hour of her working day. Generally, candidates for the position of re-care coordinator are individuals who are patients in your practice—people you know, and people who know people in your community. Often, these individuals are moms who need to get out of the house a few hours a week or people who are just simply burned out on watching Oprah and Dr. Phil.

Your new re-care coordinator will come in three days a week, from four to seven p.m. or from three to six p.m., to call people and remind them to get back into the re-care system. This fills up a major "bleeding point" in most dental practices—patients who simply fall out of the re-care system for whatever reason.

Your re-care coordinator ought to be able to enroll at least five patients a day for hygiene appointments during the three or four hours a day they work. Pay your re-care coordinator $10 an hour, and an additional $1 for each patient who makes an appointment *and shows up*. You're spending about $100 a week on your new re- care coordinator, but you're supercharging your hygienist's schedule. Your hygienist now has the maximum number of people to care for, and to whom she can present thousands of dollars of new treatment.

Take the time to train your re-care coordinator; explain exactly what you want from her. As a result, you'll get to do more dentistry without churning more patients. And no one else other than your treatment coordinator has to sell, because everybody else is playing his or her specific role.

YOU'RE SUPERCHARGING YOUR HYGIENIST'S SCHEDULE.

One more point about the re-care system before we conclude this chapter. *Aim for one hundred percent pre-*

appointments before your patients leave. Get them back into the computer immediately—don't let them out of the system. This is another "bleeding point" in the practice. Make sure that everybody gets a card one month before an appointment, a call two weeks before, and then a call forty-eight hours in advance of the appointment. If you've got people who say, "I don't know what my schedule is going to be," simply be proactive with them. Have your re-care coordinator say, "Your next appointment is three (or four or six) months from today, the same day and time. We'll keep you in the system. Call us and make a change if you need to, but we'll hold this appointment for you for now."

By getting them into the system automatically, and by contacting them three times—one month, two weeks, and then forty-eight hours prior to their next re-care appointment—you are showing your patients that you are serious about them showing up on time. This dramatically reduces the number of broken and cancelled hygiene appointments. And you don't have to make it all that easy for them to change appointments once they are made. But that's up to you.

Keep a short call list or a wish list handy for your appointment coordinator. These are individuals who would be happy to come in at a given day and time, if such appointments open up. That way, if those slots suddenly open, you've got people on the short call list who can fill them immediately.

Now, your practice runs this way:

- The re-care coordinator comes in ten hours a week and makes the calls.

- The appointment coordinator makes sure that your hygienist's time is always used to the maximum.

- Your hygienist has an hour to do her hygiene work and to do the patient education that you now want her to do.

- You come in for five minutes and confirm the case.

- Your hygienist then turns the patient over to the treatment coordinator, who arranges payment options and makes plans for the next treatment appointment, if necessary.

- You perform the dentistry, knowing that everybody else in your office is perhaps even more dedicated to keeping you working than you are!

- And then when your patient's work is finished, the patient goes directly to re-care.

This is the way truly successful dentists make huge amounts of money—they've got everybody in the office totally invested in making sure that the work is flowing and that everybody is doing his or her job. Now you know exactly what you should be doing with your dental hygienist—you want to have her serving as the linchpin of patient education in your office, because when she generates more work, far more money flows to your bottom line, perhaps as much as half a million dollars a year. And those are numbers that will put a smile on any dentist's face.

Take Your Practice to the NextLevel:

1. The more you allow your dental hygienist to do his or her real job—cleaning teeth and providing education to your patients—the less selling you'll have to do and the more dentistry you'll get to practice. Whatever your hygienist says, nod and say "OK." Then say, "Let me take a look and confirm." Reconfirming your hygienist's analysis adds credibility to what he/she says, which increases credibility for your entire team.

2. Your hygienist can and should be a profit center and the cornerstone of the dental care delivery system in your office. When you add credibility to your hygienist by confirming his/her findings, your patients begin to listen to your entire team and respect them as a knowledgeable, well-respected unit.

3. If you give your hygienist enough time and a large enough bonus, he or she will radically increase the profitability of your practice.

4. A re-care coordinator will fill the empty places in your hygienist's schedule and keep your best patients from "slipping through the cracks." Have your coordinator run the report of patients who have not been in for their 6-month recall visit, and pay them for every patient they put back into the schedule who shows up.

Chapter 5

Why Your Team Hates You

THERE'S A WONDERFUL Peanuts cartoon where Charlie Brown is discussing with Linus who exactly in Charlie Brown's life loves him. Charlie Brown can't think of anybody. Then he remembers Snoopy.

"Snoopy doesn't count," Linus reminds him. "You feed him.

He *has* to love you."

I tell this story now to illustrate the point that some dentists don't realize exactly how their team members feel about them. The unfortunate reality is that team members in many dental offices have feelings toward their dentist-employers that range from cordial dislike to outright animosity. There are many reasons for this, as we shall see in this chapter, but the obvious point is that it's hard to have a dental office create huge amounts of success and wealth for the dentist when his team can't stand him.

Some of my clients have been shocked to discover that their team members don't like or respect them nearly as much as they had previously thought. As in the Peanuts cartoon, these dentists often fail to realize that their team members are beholden to the dentist for their jobs and their livelihoods. Workers tend to treat their boss with at least a minimal amount of respect, since he or she is signing their paychecks. But does that grudging respect, often insincere, really translate into the team liking the dentist, wanting to go all out for him, ready to go that extra mile?

> **THE UNFORTUNATE REALITY IS THAT TEAM MEMBERS IN MANY DENTAL OFFICES HAVE FEELINGS TOWARD THEIR DENTIST-EMPLOYERS THAT RANGE FROM CORDIAL DISLIKE TO OUTRIGHT ANIMOSITY.**

As long as you're writing checks, people will have a higher affinity to you. But an affinity based strictly on paychecks is simply not sufficient for the kind of relationships you need with your team in order to maximize the effectiveness—and the profitability—of your practice.

In this chapter, I'd like to explore the sometimes edgy relationships that may exist between dentists and their teams. Then I want to show you how to transform the nature of your relationships with each of your team members so that the office operates in the smoothest, most frictionless way possible.

I'd like to bring back from Chapter 1 our old friend Larry Laserguy, D.D.S. Like some dentists, Larry has an often uneasy relationship with his team. I'd like to take you inside Larry's practice and show you the nine reasons why his team doesn't love him.

1. Broken Agreements and Promises.

Larry has the nasty habit of hiring individuals to do one job but then making them do something else, often something they don't want to do. Larry's dental hygienist is frequently asked to jump on the phones when no one else can do it. His dental assistant frequently has to work the front desk whenever the front desk person (more about that title later) doesn't show up for work, takes an extremely extended coffee break or lunch, or otherwise isn't available. Larry made these individuals promises back when he hired them, but cash-flow concerns or a too-busy schedule has prevented him from seeing those agreements through.

Another classic example of a broken agreement is Larry's promise to all of his new hires to give them a review in ninety days with the possibility of a pay raise if they have done well to that point. The ninety-day mark comes and goes, but that promised review never materializes, and neither does the raise. Was Larry being sincere when he made the promise to give a review in ninety days? Most likely. It's just that he never made a note to himself in his date book to keep that commitment. And then the team member never brought it up again, so it completely slipped Larry's mind. At least until the next time he hires somebody and makes the same promise, a promise that he breaks again and again.

How do Larry's team members feel when they have been promised a review and a possible raise, and neither materializes? As you can imagine, they feel quite bad about it. They're not going to say anything to Larry, because they don't want to risk their jobs.

Instead, they will feel resentful, and they will act resentfully toward Larry. Since they see that Larry is doing the minimum for them, they will do the minimum for Larry. Their attitude rapidly disintegrates from "I'm going to do the best job I can" to "I'm gonna take the money and run." Can Larry really blame them?

2. Larry Manages by Emotion Rather Than by Results.

Larry has a tendency to base his management style, on any given day, on a variety of factors that have little to do with making an office run well. If he had a good night at home with his wife, Larry is likely to be all smiles in the morning, treating everybody with backslapping glee. If he had a fight with his wife, or if his accountant called and told him that his cash flow wasn't where it needed to be, or if one of his kids made yet another demand for a new 3 Series convertible (or a new Boxster, given the nature of Larry's kids), then it's going to be a rough day at the office for the whole team. Larry is going to be barking orders, making incessant demands, and generally treating everybody shabbily. Larry leads by emotion, rather than giving people clear guidelines, clear responsibilities, and a clear sense of what constitutes acceptable results.

3. Larry's Got a New Long-Term Plan Every Two Weeks.

Larry has a real penchant for seminars, motivational tapes, books, and other "tools" for improving his practice. Frequently, Larry will take a Friday off to attend a seminar on how to improve some aspect of his dental practice. He'll get all jazzed up over the weekend about these ideas, and then come in Monday morning with a brand new set of management tools, slogans, trinkets, or who knows what to motivate (and sometimes terrorize) the team. Of course, by Tuesday or Wednesday, Larry's ardor for these new innovations has cooled, and by the end of the week, it's back to business as usual.

As a result, no one in the office takes it seriously when Larry enthusiastically institutes a brand new set of procedures on Monday morning, because everybody knows they'll be gone with the wind by Friday afternoon. Larry, for his part, can't understand why his team members never buy into these great ideas. How can he make money, he asks himself, when he's got a bunch of people allergic to change working for him?

4. Larry is Either Too Controlling or Too Lax.

You could say that Larry has a split personality. Sometimes, he micromanages everything that happens in the office, making sure that everybody is busy doing something, regardless of whether that "something" actually benefits the bottom line. When people see Larry in that frame of mind, they snap to attention and start looking busy. The office takes on the energy (and fear) of an Army base, where everybody is either saluting or painting something. When Larry gets in his super-controlling mode, nothing of any importance gets done in the office. People are too busy looking busy, too scared that he might turn and snap at them.

At other times, Larry is simply too lax. His team whispers that he has no backbone and that he actually wants his team to lead him, instead of the other way round. He doesn't deal with troublesome situations or quarrelsome people. He doesn't have the guts to confront the team member who is behaving badly, showing up late, stealing from the office, picking fights with everybody else, or just generally making a dreadful nuisance of himself or herself. Everybody wishes Larry would step up and fire that person, but Larry is simply too afraid of confrontation. He thinks in terms of scarcity—the crummy employee he has is better than nothing, and how on earth can he hope to find somebody who is at least as minimally as competent as this person, despite all the trouble that he or she causes?

As a result of Larry's lax nature, unless he is in his hyper- control mode, the office is really run by the strongest personality in the suite. In Larry's office, it happens to be Anita, his strong-willed appointment coordinator. She is the most feared person in the office, making every decision from hiring to salaries, from choosing vendors to installing new technologies. She's running a multi-million-dollar dental practice, with no business training and not even a great deal of aptitude for the job. But Larry is too scared to stand up to her, and so is everyone else in the office. No wonder Larry's team hates him. They want an office to be run by a leader, and they want the leader to be Larry and no one else.

5. Larry Lives in a World Where it is Better to Look Good Than to be Real.

His team cannot stand what they consider his addiction to inauthenticity. They all know what he drives—they all see that fully loaded 7 Series BMW in his reserved parking space right next to the elevator, while the rest of them have to park in unreserved spaces further away. They all know that Larry prides himself on belonging to the best country club in town. They also know how much that car, the country club, and the whole lifestyle cost Larry. At the same time, they know that Larry refuses to give them the fifty-cent-an-hour raise that they expect, after having worked so many years at relatively low pay.

For Larry to give any one team member a fifty-cent-an-hour raise would equal about four tankfuls of gas in his Beemer over the course of the year. But does Larry pay up? Of course not. Does his team notice this? You bet.

6. Larry Always Has to be Right.

"Doctor knows best," is Larry's philosophy. He blames everybody else in the office when things go wrong, when he isn't making as much as his buddies at the club, or when anything happens that meets with his disapproval. And Larry is a very hard person to please. He frequently vents his frustration and is upset at his team members in front of patients. This really drives Larry's team nuts. It's bad enough that he always has to be right, and it's bad enough that he can't possibly see that the lax, careless manner in which he runs the office, and the degree to which he allows his appointment coordinator to be the real boss, is responsible for the confusion—and low profitability—of the office. If Larry didn't have to be right so often, his team might find him a little bit easier to bear.

7. Larry Treats his Patients with Respect and Patience, While he Treats his Team Like Garbage.

Larry does this because he thinks that his patients pay the bills. If only he realized that if he took proper care of his team, they would feel energized to take great care of his patients. The technical term for the way Larry's team views his relations with his patients is "sucking up." His team members feel that Larry spends so much time kissing his patients' asses that they wonder how he has any time left over to kick theirs. Larry doesn't realize that if he would only make his team number one, they would take even better care of his patients, and he'd be even more successful as a result.

8. Larry Uses Names for Jobs that Demean his Team Members.

He calls the single most valuable person in his office—the woman who steps in and handles any crisis or emergency without being asked twice and who willingly fills in at

the front desk or wherever she is needed—"the floater."
Floater? Not a lot of dignity in that term. Larry also tends
to call his front desk people "the front desk people." Are
they people? Or are they desks? Larry hasn't learned to re-
label job titles, so that people are defined by what they are
accountable for and not by where they sit. When Larry gets
around to turning his "floater" into an "MVP" and his front
desk people into appointment coordinators, re-care coordinators, insurance coordinators, and such, his employees
will have greater self-esteem and greater esteem for their
positions in his office.

9. **Larry Consistently Fails to Provide the Three
   Most Important Things a Team Member Values—
   Appreciation and Acknowledgment, Safety and
   Security, and Respect.**

Larry doesn't realize that talk isn't just cheap—it's free. It
wouldn't kill him to say a few appreciative or thoughtful
words to the people who bust their butts on his behalf. But
he never can bring himself to do so. He keeps everybody in
the office running so scared that they have no sense of job
security. Larry's pretty quick to threaten to fire people—
behind their backs, because he believes that an office that
runs scared runs well. (Larry's wrong, of course, but you
and I know that.)

And when it comes to respecting the team members…
fuggetaboutit. Larry has the inability to control his tongue,
whether he is criticizing a team member in front of other
team members or in front of patients.

When an employer consistently fails to provide these three basic desires—appreciation and acknowledgment, safety and security, and respect—there's only one thing left for a team member to hang onto. And that's money. Once again, Larry unwittingly instigates in his people an attitude of "take the money and run." He isn't even aware of the things that come out of his mouth, because he figures that he's the boss, and whatever he says has to be right. Poor Larry. He just doesn't get it.

That line from Cool Hand Luke—"What we have here is a failure to communicate"—applies to Larry's office in spades. There's a lack of timely, efficient communication. Nobody knows what's flying. When there are important changes, news comes only through gossip. Information travels quickly—and inaccurately—from team member to team member. Everybody resents the fact that Larry doesn't take the time to inform them in a structured way about things that are going on in the office.

If Larry were wise, he could solve this problem by holding twice-monthly team meetings with everyone present, monthly department lunches, and daily morning meetings. That way, he can get all the information out to his team members without playing the "telephone game," where the information is usually totally garbled by the time it reaches the end of the line.

WHEN AN EMPLOYER CONSISTENTLY FAILS TO PROVIDE THESE THREE BASIC DESIRES—APPRECIATION AND ACKNOWLEDGMENT, SAFETY AND

SECURITY, AND RESPECT—THERE'S ONLY ONE THING LEFT FOR A TEAM MEMBER TO HANG ONTO. AND THAT'S MONEY.

To summarize these nine points, it all comes down to a lack of integrity on Larry's part.

Integrity means being true to your word. It means that people will follow where you lead, because they know they can trust you to keep the commitments that you make. When I work with doctors, I share with them the simple fact that their team members will only trust them in the future to the extent that they have kept their word to their team members in the past. The better a doctor is at not keeping his word, the less power he has as a leader.

My clients often feel a sense of despair at this point. They realize that they have been guilty of making promises they haven't kept—like promising reviews, rewards, raises, bonuses, and the like. They may have wanted to keep those promises, but their inadequate cash flow or lack of time prevented them from doing so. Again, as the expression goes, green goes with everything. The more money you are bringing in, the easier it is to be generous with your team.

In the past, doctors may have shifted people from the position for which they were hired to tasks they really didn't want to do, and those doctors didn't really care how much it bothered their employees that they had to perform tasks outside their basic job description.

My clients have come to realize that they spent enormous amounts of time and effort buttering up the patients when they should have been treating their teams as number one. They realize that speaking harshly and critically of a team member in front of a patient or other team members has been a regular part of their approach to doing business, and now they see that this approach is counterproductive.

They realize that they have been too controlling, micromanaging and redirecting the efforts of team members, when their team members know exactly what to do and how to do it. Or they have been too lax, giving away far too much power to a team member who is neither trained for nor appropriate for handling so important a role.

They further realize that they have failed to fire the "problem child" in their office—the individual whose inappropriate behavior sets the whole office on edge, destroys morale, and encourages other team members to behave badly as well.

My clients feel a momentary sense of despair at this juncture, because they suddenly realize that the tongue in the shoe does not match the tongue in the mouth—they've said things would change, but they never caused a change. They might have had good intentions, but they lacked the ability, the time, the knowledge, or the structure to make necessary changes. The bottom line: They didn't keep their word.

So what do they do now?

Here's the good news: *It's not nearly as hard as you think to restore your team's trust in you.*

Restoring trust requires doctors first to realize that eighty percent of the problems in their offices come from promises that they made... and broke. As a result, their word has no value. They can't create a new future, and they can't solve the problems from the past. They are just stuck.

IT'S NOT NEARLY AS HARD AS YOU THINK TO RESTORE YOUR TEAM'S TRUST IN YOU.

So what do you have to do to get your team completely on your side? Before I answer that question, I want to explain how I learned about the value of integrity. To put it simply, I learned it the hard way. I was running a consulting firm, and I hired a business coach to show me how to take my firm to the next level. After a number of sessions, he said to me, "Gary, you don't keep your word. How can you expect your business to grow if you don't keep your word? All your business practices are fine, but you lack integrity."

I was stung by his words. "What are you talking about?" I asked. "Give me an example of where I'm not true to my word!"

"You're late all the time," my coach said.

"*That's* a breach of integrity?" I asked, amazed. I couldn't believe it! "I'm late maybe five minutes every so often. Why is that such a big deal?"

"If you don't keep your word all the time," my coach said, "you are devaluing your word. And nobody's going to trust you. Being five minutes late for meetings just doesn't work. It's an insult to the people with whom you are meeting, because you're essentially telling them that your time is far more important than theirs."

I didn't like where this was going, as you can imagine.

"I want to make an agreement with you," he continued. "From now on, every minute you're late, it's going to cost you a hundred dollars. We'll reconcile at the end of the month. Deal?"

"Deal," I said, laughing, and we shook hands.

Little did I know that my coach was serious.

At the end of the month, I arrived at my session—a couple of minutes late, I must confess—and my coach said, "You owe me thirty-five hundred dollars. You were late a total of thirty-five minutes this month. I'm not going to work with you any longer unless you pay me."

I couldn't believe what I was hearing. "I thought we were just kidding about that!" I exclaimed.

"I was completely serious," my coach said, "and we shook hands on it. Gary, we made an agreement. You've got to honor it." I did what just about anybody would do in that position. I walked out. I didn't need him to fine me for being late. Who did he think he was? I could do just fine building my consulting practice *without his help*.

But the next two or three weeks were pure torture for me. I just couldn't stand the fact that he was right and I was wrong. I hadn't kept my word.

I scheduled a new session with my coach and went back to his office, carrying a check for thirty-five hundred dollars.

"You've done a very smart thing," my coach said. "You're going to see that this thirty-five hundred dollars will turn into millions."

He was right. It has, for myself and for my clients. I keep my agreements, and I expect my clients to keep their agreements with me. By learning to keep their agreements, my clients discover that people listen to them much more carefully. They are able to enroll their team members and their patients (and their family members, too!) in new, healthy agreements, because everyone in their lives now recognizes that these individuals will keep their word.

A lot of people in our society think that they can make more money by scamming, trying to get over on people, trying to hustle or take advantage. The reality is that you have a much better time—and you make a heck of a lot more money—when you color within the lines. That's the foundation of integrity.

Let's return now to the question of how you develop trust with your team members, especially in situations where trust was lacking in the past. You start by drawing a line in the sand. You tell your team, "The past is over. We're going to start fresh with a clean sheet of paper."

Here's what you do: You sit down with each member of your team and you listen, without judgment. Here's what you say: "I want to have a genuine conversation with you, a conversation that's different from any we've ever had in the past. I want to know if there's anything that affects our relationship, anything from the past, any agreement I haven't kept, that keeps you from being fully engaged and giving your absolute best."

They won't tell you everything, and there may be nothing to tell. Yet the fact that you're taking these actions will elevate their trust in you. But they'll most likely tell you at least a few things that you might not want to hear, that you need to do differently, if you want to gain and build their trust.

Listen without judgment to the points that these individuals make. Find out what it would take to get these issues handled. And then do whatever it takes to be true to the promises that you made in the past, broken promises of which you are being reminded now, or the promises that you are making in this conversation. Tell your people that you want to take responsibility for keeping your word and for the fact that you haven't kept your word in the past. Remember that they are going to be sharing with you their reality, not yours. Your mission here is to get the facts.

Until you've got your entire team confronting the problems about how *you've* been dealing with them, you simply can't create a new future. You'll be like Larry Laserguy, all revved up from that seminar he took last Friday, unable to enroll any of his people in the changes he'd like to effect, simply because they don't have any reason to believe him. You are going to do it differently. You are going to take responsibility for the broken promises of the past, and you're going to take responsibility for keeping your word in the future.

If you want your team to give you their best, then you've got to play straight with them. No more broken agreements. If you promise to show up on time and you're late, acknowledge when you're late. Don't just let it slide.

Don't criticize your team members in front of each other or in front of patients. Treat your team members right, and they will end up treating your patients so well that you won't have to put so much effort into diplomacy instead of dentistry. If there's a problem child in the office, fire that person immediately. Normally I don't recommend firing people, but in this case, you've got to do it, for the good of all.

Don't let your office manager—or your dental assistant, or even your hygienist—run the office any longer, if that has been going on. Initially, these strong-willed individuals may be afraid of me, or of any good consultant, because they fear losing power. Part of my job is to reassure them that things will be fine for them even if they're not in a power position. You've got to be the boss. We'll talk more about how to make that happen in later chapters, but this is the way you've got to start thinking.

Another key point: Stop scheduling the team member—schedule the position. Instead of micromanaging what everybody in your office is doing, instead create the positions of treatment coordinator, appointment coordinator, re-care coordinator, and so on, as we have discussed and as we will discuss further in later chapters, and make sure that someone is filling each of those positions every hour. Make sure that people have specific tasks for which they are accountable, goals they are to reach, structures in place for helping them reach those goals, and accountability measures so that *you*—and they—can see if they are doing their jobs. And then turn them loose. Give them the responsibility they need and the trust they need, so they know that you—and the rest of the team—know that they'll do their jobs properly.

Along these lines, set up accountabilities that are tied to tangible results. Put a structure in place, a piece of paper, a computer program, some way of tracking what they are supposed to do. Then monitor the statistics—how much is being sold, produced, collected? How many people are seated on time every day? Third, establish a process by which each individual will accomplish what he or she is supposed to do. And then step back and let them do what they need to do.

In so doing, you will shift their thinking about money from "He treats me so badly, I'm just going to take the money and run" to "I wouldn't go somewhere else, even for more money." My clients frequently have lower salary costs, because they are careful to provide their team members with the appreciation and acknowledgment, respect, and security *they actually value more than money*.

Don't be afraid to share the numbers with your team members. Let them know how you're doing. Forty percent of the doctors who hire me initially won't share their numbers with anyone else in the office. This kind of secrecy is counterproductive. It's like going to a ball game without a scoreboard. Everybody needs to know exactly how they are doing, relative to rational expectations for their position.

Give up the idea of "doctor knows best." Keep in mind that your team members need a measuring stick. They need a means of course correction if they're not getting done what they need to accomplish. Fix the process; stop blaming the people.

Try to see things from their point of view. Right now, most dentists have only one view of their office—top down. They don't think even for a moment about what it's like to work at any of the other positions on the team. As part of my training to work with dentists, I spent weeks in dental offices, seeing what everybody does and how they're treated. I sat next to the hygienist. I didn't scrape teeth, but I sat beside her and watched what she goes through. I sat next to the assistant on the high speed, when the dentist was doing four wisdom teeth extractions. I don't like the sight of blood, but I sure did get to see their experience.

GIVE UP THE IDEA OF "DOCTOR KNOWS BEST."

I've sat next to insurance coordinators in dental offices, watching them as they are on the phone with insurance companies. Most dentists have no idea what it takes for a team member to get the appropriate information from an insurance company. As a result, they underestimate the amount of time that a job takes, and then they become annoyed when their team members aren't getting done what they need to get done in a timely fashion. Try to see what life is like from the perspective of your team members. It will most likely be an eye-opening experience for you.

Expect to be tested. Your team won't know initially whether your new approach to integrity and trust is the wave of the future or a one-day wonder. Expect them to hold you to this word that you're now promising to keep. Expect them to challenge you if you aren't living up to your promises. Above all, be patient with them. They had to live with the "old" you for a long time! Don't expect them to act anything other than wary and mistrustful at first. They'll come around. And if any of them don't come around, if any of your team members prefer to wallow in their misery instead of getting with the new program, don't worry about it. They'll fire themselves. If they're unhappy working in a productive, upbeat, successful office, they'll leave to find a place where the company loves misery. You won't even have to fire the problem people. They really will fire themselves.

To come back to the title of this chapter, team members

hate dentists who don't keep their word. Team members hate dentists who lack integrity and who cannot be trusted. If you are willing to display the humility that it takes to acknowledge that your word has not been worth all that it should have been in the past, if you're willing to sit down and really listen to your team members and find out what promises have not been kept, and if you are willing to walk your talk and act in a trustworthy manner, displaying the kind of integrity that they want you to demonstrate as the captain of the ship, your team will treat you with respect. Your office will be a much happier place in which to work or receive services. And you'll discover that it's not your patients who really pay your bills. It's actually your team that will be generating the growth of your practice... and your income, by taking the best possible care of your patients on your behalf. Your newfound commitment to integrity and trust will demonstrate itself in a highly dramatic fashion... in your bottom line.

Take Your Practice to the NextLevel:

1. Practicing integrity is the key to the successful practice of dentistry. Integrity doesn't matter if you aren't aspiring to something great. The truth is that life works, whether you keep your promises or not. However, if you're aiming for something awesome—like having an amazing profitable business, perhaps—integrity matters! So keep your promises to your staff, patients, friends, and family. When's the best time to restore your integrity? RIGHT NOW!

2. For one week, keep your promise with two specific things each day. For example, if you say you will be home at 5pm, be home at 5pm. If you tell your child you'll be at their practice or rehearsal at a certain time, be there when you said you would, with a smile and positive attitude to boot.

3. Integrity means keeping your promises to your team with regard to salary, benefits, reviews, and any other commitments you make. They deserve appreciation, acknowledgement, safety, security, and respect. Your team, not just your patients, are the cornerstone of your successful practice. You can't have a successful dental practice alone—you have to have a dependable team. It's

important to remember that the staff will only be as dependable as you are. If you don't keep your promises to them, they have no reason to keep their promise to you to serve your customers.

If your team isn't performing up to their full potential, examine the ways in which you may be unconsciously cutting your own support system out from under you. What have you promised and not delivered? Have there been review dates that were not met? If so, restore your word today.

When it comes to acknowledging the contributions of your team, always go the extra mile. Write a thank you card to each one of your team members to acknowledge them for all the things they do right. It's also important to say these things out loud to your team—even if it means reading off the card! If you want love and respect you got to give it away. Swing out and do it today.

Chapter 6

There's a Fortune in Your Storage Closet

DENTISTS ALWAYS WANT to know the key to closing big cases. The simple fact is that you can't close big cases if you don't present them. I often ask dentists what is the biggest case they ever closed. The typical response is $15,000 to $20,000. How did you do it? I ask. Invariably, it turns out that the dentist didn't do anything. A patient simply came in and said, "Do my whole mouth."

So then I ask the dentist, "What's the most you've ever presented, educated about, and closed?" The answer is in the $3,000 to $5,000 range. Dentists who don't have a method in place for presenting comprehensive cases cannot close them.

The key to closing big cases is to know how to have your entire office involved in the selling process—so you can be chairside, doing the work that's the most interesting and lucrative for you, all day long.

Most dentists despise anything to do with the concept of selling. They see themselves, and correctly so, as health professionals, and they regard selling as dirty, disreputable, and somehow beneath them. The problem is, if you don't sell, you don't work. Most dental practices plod along in a mediocre fashion because the dentists simply don't realize how important it is to know how to sell.

Alternatively, some dentists take an overly aggressive approach to sales. They hammer their patients and annoy them so much that the dentist is the last person on earth the patient ever wants to see. Some hygienists tell me that their patients want to avoid any contact with the dentist while they are getting their teeth cleaned. The patients actually ask the hygienist to sneak them out of the office before the dentist gets there. That shows you the extent to which dentists who are overly aggressive in their sales practices upset their patients and lose sales.

> **IRONICALLY, IF YOU PUT THE PROCEDURES IN THIS CHAPTER INTO PLACE, YOU WON'T HAVE TO DO MUCH—OR ANY—OF THE SELLING.**

I want to propose a happy medium, a situation in which you feel comfortable enough with the sales process so that you are able to generate the huge amounts of income that we talked about earlier in this book. Ironically, if you put the procedures in this chapter into place, you won't have to do much—or any—of the selling. Your team will be doing it for you, allowing you to practice the kind of dentistry you want to practice, while making the kind of money you may never have dreamt that you could make.

Most dentists—and most people, for that matter—think

about sales as a process of forcing other people to do things against their will and not necessarily in their best interests. That's a form of sales, certainly, but unfortunately, the entire world of sales is tainted by that perception. Those tactics may be appropriate on a third-rate used car lot, but the fact is that you can sell with dignity and respect for yourself, your patient, and the practice of dentistry. Let me show you how.

Let's review what we've discussed already about the nature of my approach to building a dental practice. Your re-care coordinator will be making sure that your hygienist has a completely booked schedule. Your appointment coordinator makes sure that the calendar is adhered to and that if patients cancel at the last moment, other patients from the "wish list" or short-call list are called and take those appointment times that otherwise would have gone empty. The hygienist gets a full hour with each patient, in order to perform her work to the highest professional degree, and then she educates the patient in terms of what problems she sees and what dental work is necessary in order to treat those problems. She'll be putting up at least four pictures on the intraoral camera so that the patient—and you—can see exactly what needs to be done.

Only at that point will you step into the hygienist's room, not to slice and dice the patient with high pressure sales tactics, but simply to confirm the work that the hygienist has suggested. You'll answer any questions the patient might have, and then *you leave the room*.

With you moving on to do more important things with your time, the hygienist finishes up her session with the patient and turns the patient over to the treatment coordinator, who will go over the nature of the treatment, answer concerns and questions, and make agreements with regard to time and money. How much selling did you have to do in that paradigm?

Not much at all.

Selling really *isn't* your business. Setting up a system in your office by which sales can happen easily—that's your responsibility.

> **SELLING REALLY ISN'T YOUR BUSINESS.**
> **SETTING UP A SYSTEM IN YOUR OFFICE**
> **BY WHICH SALES CAN HAPPEN EASILY**
> **THAT'S YOUR RESPONSIBILITY.**

The key to this process working is to allow your treatment coordinator to have a dedicated space in which to hold these extremely important conversations with the patients. This point is so important that I want to repeat it, because I don't want you to miss it. You must give your treatment coordinator a dedicated space where she will do the selling for you, in a dignified and entirely honorable manner.

Most dentists respond, "I simply don't have the space!" In ninety-nine percent of the cases, that's just not true. There's often a corner of the front office area where the team stores those big five-gallon water bottles. That area could be cleaned out and you can put in movable partitions to create a dedicated treatment coordinator space. There's also your office, which you occupy only about ten percent of the time. You'll be in there even less as you spend increasing amounts of lucrative time chairside. The treatment coordinator could easily set up shop there.

Another approach is to take a second look at your storage closet. Most dental offices have storage closets that are filled not with supplies but with old junk that no one has the interest—or often the authority—to remove. What about your office? Do you have a "storage closet" with ancient computer gear that no one on the planet could possibly use? Might it be filled with the old office furniture that somehow never got dumped, or other large, bulky pieces of equipment that are no longer part of your practice?

If so, that storage closet that could be transformed into a treatment coordinator's office is costing you hundreds of thousands of dollars a year until you clean it out and use it at its highest level of efficiency.

Let's take a look at what goes on in that office, and then let's take a look at how it should appear.

The first thing to note about the treatment coordinator's space, whether it is a newly formed cubicle somewhere in your office area, your own office, or the storage closet that you are transforming, is that *no one else should use it under any circumstances for any other purpose.* This is not a place for team members to go make personal phone calls. This is not a place for your assistant to fill out charts. This space has to be one hundred percent dedicated to the use of the treatment coordinator. It's going to cost you far too much money to allow it to be used for any other purpose at any time.

So lay down the law—this space belongs to the treatment coordinator, or the secondary treatment coordinator when your treatment coordinator's out of the office. The space is inviolate and cannot be used by any other person for any other purpose at any time.

By now, in our new process, the hygienist has walked the patient from her room to the treatment coordinator's office. *At this moment, the patient's emotional attachment to getting the dental work done is at its highest.* Keep in mind that people buy based on their emotions and then justify their purchases based on logic (that's how Larry Laserguy leased his big Beemer, right?). **If patients leave before they have made agreements about the nature of the work to be performed, the time or times when that work will be performed, and the cost and method of payment for that work, their emotional connection to getting the work done will diminish rapidly… and then you've lost them.**

I'm not suggesting that you hammer people, or have your treatment coordinator hammer people on your behalf. I am suggesting strongly that your closing ratio will collapse if you are not getting agreements at the time when emotions are the strongest.

When the patient gets home, if these agreements have not already been put in place, the spouse might say, "It's not worth that kind of money—that dentist is a scammer. I don't want to spend it. It doesn't hurt, does it?" And other sorts of things will intervene to diminish the likelihood that the patient will return to get the work done.

> **YOUR CLOSING RATIO WILL COLLAPSE IF YOU ARE NOT GETTING AGREEMENTS AT THE TIME WHEN EMOTIONS ARE THE STRONGEST.**

So it's the role of your treatment coordinator to get agreements while the patient's emotional attachment to getting the work done is at its peak. The treatment coordinator will first go over the nature of the treatment with the patient. The treatment coordinator needs to recognize that patients often don't listen to dentists, because when dentists speak, patients are dealing with their own fears about pain and expense. On top of that, dentists often use terms that make a lot of sense to the dentist, but make no sense to the patient. So it's up to your treatment coordinator to explain the nature of the treatment in lay person's terms, go over the questions, concerns, and fears of the patient, and make sure that the patient understands exactly what is necessary.

For example, the dentist might take a quick look in the patient's mouth and say, "You need root planing and scaling." First, this language is frightening to the patient. It sounds painful, it sounds unpleasant, and it sounds expensive. What the dentist has done—and dentists do this all the time—is to skip the nature of the problem and instead proceed directly to the proposed solution. Why do dentists think primarily in terms of solutions? Because they think that solutions put money in their pockets.

If a dentist sees a mouth in which root planing and scaling is necessary, the dentist knows that this is a case he is likely to close for about eight hundred dollars. Dentists are sometimes thinking on a subconscious level about exactly where that money is going—to help defray a mortgage payment, a car payment, an alimony payment, or some other specific, and often overwhelming, financial need. In other words, dentists aren't always thinking about patient care. They're thinking about the many responsibilities they have, including paying their own bills. That's not the best mindset with which to win the trust of a patient.

By the way, the hygienist and the dentist should never be talking about money and insurance. Remember that the patient is in a very vulnerable situation in that dental chair and won't be able to focus on information about money and insurance at that time. In any event, money and insurance are the wrong things for hygienists and dentists even to be thinking about. Your focus, and your hygienist's focus, should be on getting the patient well. If the patient asks you about the cost of treatment, your only response should be, "My job is to tell you what's happening. My treatment coordinator will discuss with you everything to do with money."

THE HYGIENIST AND THE DENTIST SHOULD NEVER BE TALKING ABOUT MONEY AND INSURANCE.

The treatment coordinator therefore needs to remember that the doctor was probably speaking in a language the patient could not comprehend—or probably even hear straight. The treatment coordinator also has to recognize that there is a lot of fear going on in that hygienist's room. To put it simply, *everybody's afraid*. The *dentist* is afraid that if he doesn't close the case, he won't be able to meet his many financial obligations. The *patient* is afraid that it's going to hurt and cost a lot. The *hygienist* is afraid that she will lose credibility with the patient if the dentist contradicts her suggestions that are based on the office's agreed-upon standard of care.

By now, you've read enough of this book to know that you've got to think about life from the patient's point of view and not just from your own. Of course, your job is not to be Dr. Phil. Your job is to be a dentist., and this means that the psychology—and financial aspects—of your patients' situation shouldn't be your concern. It's up to the treatment coordinator to spell out exactly what you were talking about, if you weren't clear enough when you were telling the patient what was necessary and why.

In our earlier example, your treatment coordinator ought to explain root planing and scaling in this manner: "We're going to meticulously deep clean your gums, removing all the bacteria that eats away at your bone. If you don't do this, you'll lose your teeth. Gum disease is a silent killer of teeth. Many people come to us when it's too late, when gum disease has already done its work, and by then we can't stabilize the condition. Everybody wants to be able to eat crusty bread or corn on the cob their whole life. If we get your mouth really clean in this manner, you'll be able to enjoy complete confidence that you'll keep your teeth."

This is what I mean by addressing the dental situation in terms that the patient can understand.

At this point, then, the treatment coordinator has demonstrated to the patient the value of the particular treatment the hygienist has proposed and the dentist has agreed to. Now you've got the patient saying, "I understand exactly what the treatment is! Get that nasty stuff out of my mouth!"

This brings the treatment coordinator to her next task— *to assist the patient in paying for the treatment*. Only when the patient understands the value of the treatment should you present the investment necessary for the treatment.

The treatment coordinator has established value in the mind of the patient for the treatment, and the patient has a very strong emotional attachment to getting this situation handled *right now*. The next thing for us to discuss is the role of insurance in paying for dental care.

Before the patient has even entered the treatment coordinator's office, the treatment coordinator should determine exactly how much the patient's insurance, if the patient has insurance, will cover. You want the treatment coordinator to get the patient to think of dental insurance as a benefit, not as a cure-all for the high cost of dentistry. The treatment coordinator has to get the patient away from the mindset that says that "insurance" covers everything. Instead, you want the patient to view insurance like getting a discount. You will have people saying, "What does my insurance cover? That's all I want to pay."

ONLY WHEN THE PATIENT UNDERSTANDS THE VALUE OF THE TREATMENT SHOULD YOU PRESENT THE INVESTMENT NECESSARY FOR THE TREATMENT.

Instead, your treatment coordinator should say the following: "The treatment we are discussing costs $6,000. Your insurance pays $1,000. So your out-of-pocket is only

$5,000. Everybody else who comes in the office who doesn't have your quality of insurance has to pay $6,000."

By installing this system, and by educating the patient properly, you cause the patient to think about the care instead of the bill. That's the way you handle insurance—again, you make sure the patient sees it as a benefit and not as a panacea. This dramatically reduces broken and cancelled appointments—and also reduces complaints about your work.

At this point, it's time to share with your patient four payment options. I'll share each of them with you right now, but make sure that your treatment coordinator understands that she is not to move on from one to the next until the patient has thoroughly declined the offer currently on the table.

"Now let's talk about that $5,000," your treatment coordinator says. "If you want to pay for it in full today with cash, check, or a credit card, we'll be happy to give you a courtesy discount of five percent. So if you pay in full today, instead of paying $5,000, you would only have to pay $4750. Do you want to do it that way?"

Wait and see. People with cash love to get the discount. Whatever their response, you're starting off by establishing your best case scenario—you get paid in full *right now. Do not move on to the next option unless and until the patient rejects this first approach.*

The second option is to offer third-party financing on an interest-free basis. Yes, you'll have to pay a five to ten percent fee on that money, but it's truly worth it to you, because you get the whole payment immediately from the third-party provider. Otherwise, you get it piecemeal, and you'd have to bill to get it. If the patient defaults, you've still got their money and it's no longer your problem. It's up to the third-party finance provider to try to collect. And your patient isn't going to have to make a buying decision every time he or she walks into the office.

Here's what your treatment coordinator tells the patient: "We have another option. How about having the work done interest-free for one year? Can you afford $416.66 a month?"

Again, wait and see what the patient has to say. If the patient can handle the $416.66 a month, make the deal. Yes, you'll be paying a fee to the third-party finance provider. But you don't want to look at this in terms of losing $500 ($5000 less 10%). You want to look at it in terms of making $5500 that you otherwise never would have been able to earn.

Your treatment coordinator can actually have your patient preapproved online for third-party financing through CareCredit even before the patient steps out of hygiene. You can discuss that with your third-party finance provider.

Let's say that your patient does not want to spend the $400 a month. Then and only then, proceed to this third approach, which you will offer only to your most trustworthy patients. Here's the script for your treatment coordinator: "We could do it this way. You could pay half today, and half before we complete your case."

If the patient agrees, then the patient writes a check or gives you a credit card for $2500. You then make a written agreement with a specific date for that second payment, and then you hold the patient to that agreement when the patient returns for the work. Again, only offer this approach to patients who are reliable, trustworthy individuals. You don't want to be the bank for any other kind of person.

Let's now turn to the last resort so that you don't lose the patient, in the event that the patient turns down all three of the previous payment options. Have the treatment coordinator go back to you. The treatment coordinator will say, "The patient can't handle the case—it's way out of their budget. All of the work we've proposed is urgent, but doing something is better than doing nothing at this point. Can we split this case up over a year? Can we do $2500 through CareCredit, do this tooth and that tooth and let the rest wait for a year?"

In this case, the patient's monthly outlay would be $208.33 instead of $416.66. Here's your script for whenever the treatment coordinator asks you a question like this:

"Yes."

Any questions?

If your patient continues to object, don't coerce the patient. Go back to the original point that we made in this chapter—you are in the business of educating patients as to the problems they have and the consequences they face. If the desire not to spend the money truly outweighs the need for the dentistry, if they don't want to get the problem solved, let them go. Allow the patient the freedom to accept or decline the treatment you present. You'll have plenty of other patients on whom you can practice the kind of dentistry that you want to practice. You no longer have to come from a sense of scarcity and work with people who simply do not want to pay for the quality you want to provide.

> **ALLOW THE PATIENT THE FREEDOM TO ACCEPT OR DECLINE THE TREATMENT YOU PRESENT. YOU'LL HAVE PLENTY OF OTHER PATIENTS ON WHOM YOU CAN PRACTICE THE KIND OF DENTISTRY THAT YOU WANT TO PRACTICE.**

You—and your team—can experience a paradigm shift. Instead of *selling* dentistry, you'll have the patient *buying it.*

Now that the patient sees the value in getting the dental work performed, and now that the financial issues have been resolved, we have to deal with the patient's next important barrier to getting their treatment done—their fear of pain. This fear is the next main objection that most patients express—and only when they are asked, which is all too infrequently. Most dentists take no for an answer when they present cases and never ask patients why they're saying no. The art of sales is all about the art of understanding and handling objections. Now that you're going out of the selling business and instead having your treatment coordinator handle that task, train your treatment coordinator to ask recalcitrant patients this simple question: "What's stopping you or preventing you from getting the treatment done?" As I said, nine out of ten times, after the value has been established and the financial terms have been agreed upon, the patient will respond that it has to do with fear of pain and fear of getting his or her teeth drilled.

Your treatment coordinator should then respond as follows: "We have all the comfort measures. Dr. Chairside has the latest in numbing techniques. We'll numb you before we numb you. We'll numb you and then cover you with a blanket. You can bring in your favorite CD. You can bring your teddy bear." Whatever it takes to make the patient comfortable, within the bounds of morality and good taste, is fine. But if the patient isn't asked, the patient will never explain about his or her level of fear.

You may also want to train your treatment coordinator in the traditional sales approach to handling objections called "feel, felt, find." This means that the treatment coordinator will express her response in these terms: "I understand how you feel. A lot of our patients *felt* that way. And you'll *find*… "

This approach gives the patient the sense that he or she has been heard. It then validates the patient's feelings by acknowledging that these feelings are valid and sensible and that many other new patients in the office have shared those same feelings. Those last three magic words—"And you'll find… "—offer the patient some very good news. The news is that things are different in your dentist's office. You have the latest techniques. Your patient is thinking about experiences he or she had with a prior dentist. *We're* not like *them*. It's not like when we were kids and dental technology was in the dark ages. The main thing is for you and your treatment coordinator to recognize that when patients are expressing fear, they are *coming from the past*. That's the key to understanding your patients' fear of pain. You've got to find ways to help them focus on the present moment—that your office is conscious of the suffering that people experience in the dental chair, and that you do everything in the world to minimize those negative or painful experiences.

So far, we've discussed the nature of the conversations between the treatment coordinator and patient—how to handle insurance, how to help the patient pay for care, and how to cope with fear of dentistry. Now, let's turn to the issue of how the treatment coordinator's office should appear. The setting in which this all- important conversation between the treatment coordinator and the patient takes place must be friendly. I want to give you some specific suggestions for how to set up and decorate the office.

First, it should be set up like a living room, not like a business office. Take out the desk—you want a friendlier atmosphere. Put up "after" shots on the walls, so the patients get a sense of exactly what they can look forward to. I don't believe in "before" shots. They're just too aesthetically unpleasant. Leave the "before" shots out.

Everybody loves success stories, so frame pictures of your patients with written success stories and testimonials under the picture. Spend the money to have these photos and success stories framed beautifully. Also, you want to have articles about your community work framed beautifully, because this will humanize you. Put up pictures of your entire team, along with their outside interests. This humanizes them. Write out the vision, purpose, and values of your office. Have it printed beautifully and framed nicely on your wall as well. Have patient education materials in the room—models, computer programs, whatever it takes to show patients exactly how they will benefit from the care you prescribe.

When you've got a dedicated treatment coordinator working in a dedicated treatment coordinator space, a lot of wonderful things happen. First, your bottom line soars, because you are now getting written agreements with patients as to the nature of the case, the nature of the cost, the nature of the payment method, and the specific time or times when the work will be performed. All of my clients—and I mean all of them—experienced skyrocketing gross income as a result of the changes I am proposing for you in this chapter.

You'll be getting written agreements from your patients, unlike ninety-nine percent of your fellow practitioners. They don't have true agreements with their patients, so it's not surprising when their patients break those agreements. Keep in mind also that you are allowing your patients to have their intimate conversations about medical care, emotions, and money in a private area. Again, this room always has to be ready to receive the next patient coming out of hygiene.

On top of that, you'll be reducing flow and congestion at the front desk and making the entire office considerably more serene.

If your office manager is going to be the treatment coordinator, then she should be spending ten percent of her time managing the office and ninety percent of the time serving as treatment coordinator. For the hours when she is not present in the office, or when she is performing office managing tasks, it is up to you to designate and train a secondary treatment coordinator. You've got to have a treatment coordinator on duty all the time, every hour that your office is open. Otherwise, you'll be back to the old routine of no agreements, broken agreements, unsold cases, and accounts receivable. The way to avoid that is by scheduling the position—not the person. You've always got to have someone working as treatment coordinator all the time.

YOU'VE GOT TO HAVE A TREATMENT COORDINATOR ON DUTY ALL THE TIME, EVERY HOUR THAT YOUR OFFICE IS OPEN.

To sum up, there really is a fortune in your storage closet. That fortune will manifest itself in your appointment book—and in your bankbook—the day you turn that storage closet (or other specific space in your office) into the office for the treatment coordinator.

We started off this chapter by saying that most dentists don't like to sell and don't know how to sell. My clients, who install the procedures I've outlined for you in this chapter, are in the fortunate position of not *having* to sell. Their teams do that for them. And their teams do it beautifully.

Once you learn and install this new system, neither you, your team, or your patients will ever want to go back to the old way. Think about it: Your patient will get educated and will know exactly what's necessary. Your hygienist and assistants, and the rest of your team, will feel fulfilled. They're getting to help people, which is exactly what drove them into dentistry in the first place.

And coincidentally, you're going to get really, really wealthy; you'll work less, and have more fun and respect.

Take Your Practice to the NextLevel:

1. Give your treatment coordinator a dedicated, quiet space in which to create clear and specific agreements with patients regarding the nature of their treatment, the method of payment, and the importance of keeping appointments. For a checklist for what things you should have in your treatment room, go to my website at www.GaryKadi.com.

2. Always present treatment to the patient in terms of the value you and your team will provide. Show and discuss the problems and their consequences. Don't skip directly to the solutions, because if you do, you'll alienate the patient and your closing ratio will suffer. The patient must know the facts about their mouth before they can make an informed decision. They must see their mouth as you see it. It's the treatment coordinator's job to show them how.

3. Your treatment coordinator should provide multiple payment options to your patient one option at a time. Proper understanding and use of third-party financing is vital to the success of your practice. If you offer the first option and are greeted by an uncomfortable silence, don't move on to the second option without giving the patient a chance to answer. Instead, make your patient comfortable as you take time to discuss each of the options in depth.

Chapter 7

Turn Your Payroll into a Profit Center

IN THIS CHAPTER, we'll review the process by which you can reorganize your office so as to maximize income, job satisfaction for every member of the team, and the amount of time that you get to spend chairside performing the types of dentistry you most enjoy. But first, I want to introduce one new point: *Highly successful dentists stop viewing the salaries they pay their team members as an expense. Instead, they view salary as an investment in their own financial future.*

HIGHLY SUCCESSFUL DENTISTS STOP VIEWING THE SALARIES THEY PAY THEIR TEAM MEMBERS AS AN EXPENSE. INSTEAD, THEY VIEW SALARY AS AN INVESTMENT IN THEIR OWN FINANCIAL FUTURE.

This psychological shift is subtle and extremely important. Nobody likes expenses. In theory, if we could reduce our expenses, we tend to believe that our income will increase. Yet it's much more profitable to view the salaries you pay your team as an investment than an expense. In reality, *the more salary my clients pay, the more money they make.* That's because they have come to view many of their expenditures as investments in their practices, and they see the stunning return on investment that's possible for them and for their teams.

What is an investment? An investment is a situation where we place part of our money or time in a situation from which we expect back a decent—or even a substantial—return. My clients no longer begrudge the salaries they pay their team members, because they know that there's nothing on the stock market or in real estate (or even at the racetrack) that could possibly match the return on investment they receive from properly compensating their team members.

You'll notice that nowhere in this book have I suggested lavishing huge salaries on your team in order to motivate them. Rather, I *am* suggesting that you pay appropriate salaries combined with the extremely reasonable bonuses outlined earlier. This combination of appropriate salary plus reasonable bonuses creates a team highly motivated to make you money; to bring in new patients and return current ones; and close, insert, and arrange payment for the maximum amount of dentistry that your patients truly need. That's what happens when you view salary as an investment rather than an expense. You're investing in your own financial freedom when you set proper salary levels and proper bonus levels for every member of your team. When your net income increases as radically as that of *all* of my clients who have installed this system, you won't mind those few extra dollars in bonus money that you are paying out. You'll come to realize that the more dollars you pay in bonuses, the more thousands of dollars accrue to your own personal bottom line.

THE MORE DOLLARS YOU PAY IN BONUSES, THE MORE THOUSANDS OF DOLLARS ACCRUE TO YOUR OWN PERSONAL BOTTOM LINE.

This makes coming to work a game for my clients and then for every member of their teams, freeing them from the mindset of "I owe, I owe, it's off to work I go." In every game, each player has a specific position, a specific responsibility at that position, and accountabilities. The same thing ought to be going on in your office. You want to place people in a situation where they are playing a game, where they have a specific position, where they have specific responsibilities and accountabilities, and where it's possible to win. When your team members win, your patients, your team, and you are all happy.

So you want to begin to look at each position in your office as a separate business with accountability for managing its process and with specific results to be attained. In other words, each position must justify the investment you make in it. The amount of money you pay out to your team is now tied precisely to performance. This means that we no longer have two or three people manning the front desk, handling situations and crises as they arise. Instead, you are scheduling your team members to specific positions, and making sure that when the normal team member in that position isn't available, someone else is playing that position. For example, if a baseball team's shortstop can't play due to injury, the manager brings in someone else to play shortstop. He doesn't leave a massive hole in between second and third base. You've got to do the same thing.

For example, if Debbie is your appointment coordinator and there are practice hours when Debbie is not in the office, you've got to make sure that other people are trained to serve as appointment coordinator and serve in that position while she is out. You want to have no gaps on this team, because your patients can always exploit those gaps. Think about it this way: If there's no appointment coordinator, then no one's in charge of managing your office's time, and patients will break appointments or come late. If there's no treatment coordinator, there are no agreements about treatment and payment, which means that you end up with receivables instead of income. And so on.

LOOK AT EACH POSITION IN YOUR OFFICE AS A SEPARATE BUSINESS WITH ACCOUNTABILITY FOR MANAGING ITS PROCESS AND WITH SPECIFIC RESULTS TO BE ATTAINED.

It's vital to set targets for each team member. On a sports team, the manager or coach and the general manager have specific expectations for each player in each position. Your office ought to be the same way. Let's review examples of what those targets ought to be for your team members.

The re-care coordinator is accountable for securing at least five patients who need to get back into the re-care system during each session when she is on the phone. She is also accountable for quality assurance, by tracking the reasons patients are not returning to the practice. If she encounters former patients who do not want to come back, it is her responsibility to ask why and to inform you of those reasons. This is the least expensive and most effective way of maintaining quality control at your office. It's her job to ask the questions, and it's your job to listen to the hard truths she may present. It's also your job to fix those problems. The re-care coordinator receives an hourly salary plus a bonus of one dollar per individual whom she gets back into the re-care system and who shows up for his or her new appointment.

The appointment coordinator is accountable for meeting or exceeding the daily goal you set for each of the providers in your office—the dentists and the hygienists. It's also the responsibility of the appointment coordinator to minimize schedule changes and to assure that patients show up on time. We've already discussed how she can accomplish these things in previous chapters. Her bonus—like the bonus structures of everyone in the office—has to be rooted in what she does on a day-by-day basis. Most incentive plans that doctors employ don't work, because the goals cover too great a period of time. It's impossible to measure in any useful manner exactly how an individual performs over an entire quarter or an entire year. But we can certainly see whether a person is getting her job done on an hourly or daily basis. So we want to motivate our appointment coordinator by making sure that she knows she is responsible on an hour-by-hour and day-by-day basis for seeing that patients show up for their appointments— and show up on time.

Along these lines, I performed a study on the reasons that patients change their appointments. In my study, I learned that only fifteen percent of the changes that patients make are legitimate involving illness, a need to watch the children, car trouble, and the like. The other eighty-five percent of the reasons patients want to change their appointments are not legitimate. They simply have to do with the convenience of the patient or with the patient's desire to minimize contact with his or her dental office. Frankly, they'd rather be anywhere else. You cannot and should not stay in business to meet the whims of your patients. You don't have to make it easy for them to change their appointments, and you can train them to keep their appointments, except for those fifteen percent of the cases where the reasons for change are legitimate. This is something I show my clients precisely how to do. So to sum up, the appointment coordinator has a very clear job—and should be compensated in direct proportion to the manner in which she fulfills her responsibilities.

Let's turn now to the treatment coordinator. As we discussed earlier, the treatment coordinator is responsible for knowing the patient's insurance coverage, for offering treatment explanations in lay person's terms, listening to the concerns of the patients—and also listening for the unspoken concerns that patients have and successfully addressing them. In addition, the treatment coordinator is responsible for knowing how to use third-party financing and knowing how to get agreements for treatment. The treatment coordinator essentially serves as the liaison or case manager between the practice and the patient. The treatment coordinator receives as a bonus one percent of all cases over $500 that are presented, closed, and paid for. Many times, when I first offer this concept to dentists, they respond that it's not going to work. People won't prepay; it can't happen; it's not going to work in this office. But then they discover it does work, because it's a natural incentive for the treatment coordinator to receive a bonus for pre-payment of services. As she works to achieve that bonus, she's also working to achieve additional financial success for you. Many dentists are extremely surprised by the number of patients who accept the idea of pre-payment. The only reason these patients have never accepted it in the past is that it was never offered to them!

Next, the assistant. The dental assistant is responsible for serving the doctor beyond expectation. She must understand the verbal, assumed, and foreshadowed needs and wants of the dentist, his or her colleagues, and his or her patients. She also is in charge of ensuring what I call "time integrity" for the clinical team—she must make sure that the dentist's time is never wasted. Top offices actually have assistants directing the doctor during patient hours.

I like to use the analogy of a great restaurant. If you order a peppercorn steak, not only will the waiter in a great restaurant bring a steak knife, which is an *assumed* need, but the waiter will also bring an extra glass of water—a foreshadowed need—because peppercorn steak is hot. That simple *foreshadowing* of the typical expectations of the dinner represents the difference between good and great service. Your assistant should be providing you, your team, and your patients that same thoughtful service. You become more productive, and thus your assistant makes more money as well.

Next, we turn to the hygienist. As we have discussed, the hygienist is a catalyst for maintaining the practice standard for care. In other words, she is responsible for making sure that every patient has the opportunity to have the highest level of soft and hard tissue care and is the primary patient educator along those lines. She must be excellent at following the agreed-upon hygiene process, which includes the use of the intraoral camera on every patient. The dentist might slide—you're busy, and you've got a lot on your plate, between practicing dentistry, running the office, and maintaining your life at home. So the hygienist—not you—has the responsibility for holding you to the new standards that you have set for your office.

> **THE HYGIENIST—NOT YOU—HAS THE RESPONSIBILITY FOR HOLDING YOU TO THE NEW STANDARDS THAT YOU HAVE SET FOR YOUR OFFICE.**

Your associate is accountable for the long-term growth of the office, assuming the lion's share of evening and weekend hours—that is, if you continue to offer those hours. Let's talk for a moment about the idea of closing your doors nights and weekends. This idea actually terrifies many of my clients at first, because they can't imagine that their patients will stay with their practice if they no longer offer evening and weekend hours. In reality, few leave. You are seeking to create a practice that makes *your* life easier and in so doing allows you to serve your patients in an atmosphere of confidence and calm. Most of the kinds of patients you want to retain can and will readjust their schedules to see you on weekdays. Just about anybody whom you would like to serve can take off from work to go to the dentist. You are no longer running your practice just for the convenience of your patients. This is now a mutually beneficial relationship.

YOU ARE NO LONGER RUNNING YOUR PRACTICE JUST FOR THE CONVENIENCE OF YOUR PATIENTS. THIS IS NOW A MUTUALLY BENEFICIAL RELATIONSHIP.

You're running your practice in order to share with the patients the responsibility to maximize their dental health. So you don't have to stay open evenings and weekends if you don't want to. Incidentally, world-class team members are harder to attract to practices with night and evening hours. They're so good that they don't have to work those hours. Again, it's about catering to the needs of your team members—putting them *first*—so that you and they can offer your patients the highest and most professional standard of care.

Additionally, newer associates will be on call—not you. And they will be responsible for taking care of the children who come to your office and also to provide basic treatment. It's your job to do the highly productive cases, but you want to make sure that your associate gets some good cases as well. This will enhance your associate's growth and job satisfaction. As the associate grows with the practice, he or she will be integrated into more complex parts of the practice, like treatment planning of bigger cases and managing the office. The associate's focus should be on building a reputation of excellence and on marketing functions, such as running the website and attending community events.

Keep in mind that your sales system is built around your associate and not just around you. So be sure to integrate your associate into the new selling process that you've established for your office. That way you will maximize the efficiency of your associate and his or her use of the time.

Let's now turn to the office manager for a moment. The office manager is accountable for the morale of the team, for practice efficiency, and for statistical management. Keep in mind that every single process we have discussed can and must be measured statistically, and your office manager should devote ten percent of her total time to statistical management, team morale issues, and upholding agreements with patients with regard to appointments, payment, and other matters. This includes making sure that everyone is getting his or her proper bonus. The remaining ninety percent of the office manager's time should be devoted to patient relations. The main statistic that you want your office manager to observe: whether treatment presented is accepted at least eighty percent of the time. As we discussed earlier, this leads to a situation where your office is managed by results, not by emotion—not your emotions and not the emotions of your office manager—on any given day.

In order to assist your office manager in her statistical management, you want to establish tracking forms by position for every day that your practice is open. You've got to give your office manager the tools—and the time—to perform this basic statistical analysis, without which you cannot measure the progress of your office.

Keep in mind that everyone in your office—like everyone on the planet—craves *certainty*. People don't want to wonder if they're doing their job properly. When you put into place statistical measurements, you and your staff members no longer have to worry if they are doing their jobs well. The numbers speak for themselves. In addition, everyone leverages one another's efforts, because everyone knows how each other member of the office fits into the success of the office—and the bonus structure that each member will enjoy. This leads to what I call "productive" office gossip—everybody will know who is pulling his or her weight and who is not. The system is self-policing, and office politics are minimized. Again, people want to play a game instead of simply getting through the day. When you provide each team member with responsibilities, accountabilities, and rewards, they all know exactly what their positions are, exactly what they are responsible for, and exactly what they will get if they do their jobs especially well. This leads us to situations where the entire team is saying, "We won! Mrs. Smith accepted her treatment!" Don't laugh—that really does happen in my clients' offices.

I always like to suggest to my clients that they offer an annual team trip. Pick a number that you'd like to have the office achieve above the numbers in their incentive program, and when you hit it, send everybody to Vegas, or the Bahamas, or somewhere else that's fun. You can also tie in this trip with a fun continuing-ed program.

Your team will love it, and this will be a massive boost to your bottom line, especially if you pick a target thirty to forty percent above what you are used to making. Also, have a charity team and a community team for events in your neighborhood. People in the community will notice that you have a happy, together team, and they'll want to see what's going on that makes your office so special.

KEEP IN MIND THAT EVERYONE IN YOUR OFFICE—LIKE EVERYONE ON THE PLANET—CRAVES CERTAINTY. PEOPLE DON'T WANT TO WONDER IF THEY'RE DOING THEIR JOBS PROPERLY.

Don't forget to play the acknowledgment game. Catch people doing things right. You can put up Post-it notes that say "GREAT JOB, JENNIFER!" when the situation warrants. Read the acknowledgments that were distributed at the morning team meeting, and the person who gets the most acknowledgments over a month should win a day of beauty, or some other incentive.

Don't be afraid to post your statistics in the office for all your team to see. Accountability to each other is the easiest way to make sure that everybody is pulling his or her weight. Have a different team member be responsible for each team meeting—this increases their sense of involvement and importance, and it costs you nothing. You can also pick a different team member each quarter to send on a shopping spree. The possibilities are endless. The main point is simply to make sure that your team members share in the success of your office, and therefore will be motivated to increase that success.

Again, to summarize everything we've discussed about how to run your office on terms that provide maximum success, just keep these ideas in mind: First, turn it into a game; second, give each player specific responsibilities. Third, tie in accountabilities to those responsibilities, so that everybody knows exactly what everybody is supposed to be doing on any given day, both in terms of specific actions and in terms of financial results. And finally, provide bonuses, trips, acknowledgment, and other incentives that make the game truly worth playing for everyone in your office. When your team wins, you win.

Now you know how to revitalize your office and maximize the contributions of your team. In our next two chapters, we're going to focus on your patients. We'll discuss what you should be doing differently with your current patients, and a brand-new way to integrate new patients into your practice.

Take Your Practice to the NextLevel:

1. View salaries as an investment, not as an expense. Look at your ROI. How much money is each employee making you? And what would you do without them?

2. Look at each position in your office as a separate business with accountability for managing its processes and specific results to be attained. Have each of your team members write out the roles and responsibilities of their position. This enables you to not only see what they're accountable for, but to check into their reality. It also paves the way for a conversation about expectations and results.

3. Your team members crave certainty. They don't want to have to wonder if they're doing their jobs correctly. When you track performance statistics, your team members know exactly how well they are performing… and they also know who is letting the team down. Decide what your team is responsible for, and create a list of duties and expectations that you can both agree on. Set up how both you and they will track their progress to ensure that they are successfully meeting their performance goals. Evaluation is essential to success. For evaluation methods, go to our website at GaryKadi.com/TeamEvaluation

Chapter 8

When Patients Try Your Patience

MANY DENTISTS BELIEVE that the practice of dentistry would be absolutely wonderful… if it weren't for the patients.

Dentists face huge sources of stress in their lives. The four biggest ones: money, team, patients, and personal/family issues. So far in this book, we've begun to get a handle on the first two sources of stress—money and your team. In Chapter 3, we put cash in your pocket right now, and in subsequent chapters we discussed how to reorganize, motivate, and energize your team so that they are working with you to maximize your practice, instead of working against you, as they may have been in the past.

DENTISTS FACE HUGE SOURCES OF STRESS IN THEIR LIVES.

The great news about getting money and team issues handled, most dentists report, is that their home lives improve as well. Green truly does go with everything, and when a dentist is making more money and making it more easily, in a more relaxed and harmonious office, those good feelings come home along with the cash. My clients almost universally report that their relationships improve in direct proportion to the decrease in tension that they enjoy in their offices and in their personal finances. So an extremely important side benefit of straightening out your office is that your home life becomes much happier as well.

It's hard to put a price tag on a harmonious home. Of course, judges and divorce courts seem to have no problem dividing up the assets of unhappy ones! When you're making more money and having more fun, your relationships with your partner and your kids somehow magically fall into place.

In this chapter, I want to tackle with you the one major stressor remaining—your relationship with your patients. I want to show you a new way to relate to your patients—for you and for your team. When you implement the suggestions I'll offer you in this chapter about how to work with your patients, you will have removed the last remaining stumbling block to professional and personal serenity. So let's jump right in.

I'd like you to think of yourself as a master artist, and the painting of which you are most proud is your portrait of the Ideal Patient.

Most dentists think that they have to take their patients as they walk through the door—often irresponsible, often highly unpleasant to deal with, and often extremely slow to pay. I want to suggest a radical idea to you, and this is a concept that truly blows the minds of the dentists I work with.

You are free to create your own portrait of the Ideal Patient, and you can then work with your team to re-educate your current patients and transform them into the Ideal Patient you would prefer to treat.

YOU ARE FREE TO CREATE YOUR OWN PORTRAIT OF THE IDEAL PATIENT, AND YOU CAN THEN WORK WITH YOUR TEAM TO RE-EDUCATE YOUR CURRENT PATIENTS AND TRANSFORM THEM INTO THE IDEAL PATIENT YOU WOULD PREFER TO TREAT.

It's only fair; after all, you've become the ideal dentist, and your practice has become the ideal practice! Now let's hold your patients to an equally high standard. You can do it—after all, you're in control now, you make things happen, and your team believes in your ability to create transformations! They know how much more money they're making, they see how much more smoothly the office operates, now that you've established the principles we've talked about throughout this book. They get it. Now that you've been transformed and they've been transformed, it's time to transform the patients. So what I'd like you to do right now is take out your easel and your canvas and your smock and your palette and your brushes and create with me the Ideal Patient for your new approach to the practice of dentistry.

I like acronyms, and I want to share a simple acronym with you. You are now the *painter*. The brush—control—is in your hands. So let's use the word painter as an acronym to see your Ideal Patient coming to life on your canvas.

P—your Ideal Patient **P**ays for all treatment *before* the case is completed, leaving no balance due.

A—your Ideal Patient **A**ppreciates your dental practice, your team, and the quality of work all of you perform.

I—your **I**deal Patient understands that Insurance is a benefit and not a panacea. As we discussed earlier, your treatment coordinator will be educating your patient as to the right way to view insurance. Rather than reviewing it now, I would simply direct you back to the material in Chapter 6.

N—your Ideal Patient refers **N**ew Ideal Patients to your practice. You've ceased advertising in the Yellow Pages or the other time-honored—but unsuccessful—approaches to marketing and advertising. Instead, you can count on your Ideal Patients to tell your friends about their outstanding dentist. In fact, your patients can't wait to brag about you to their friends! And they will, because you exude certainty, caring, and control, which is what people really want.

T—your Ideal Patient **T**rusts the treatment that is presented and *accepts* all of it. I don't think any explanation is necessary on this point.

E—your Ideal Patient is **E**ducated as to the value of dentistry. Your Ideal Patient "gets it." He or she understands the paramount importance of achieving and maintaining outstanding dental health both now and for the future. You're no longer dealing with people who view dentistry as an intrusion in their lives but instead view it as very good fortune that they get to take the very best possible care of themselves with you in control of the situation.

And finally,

R—your Ideal Patient **R**espects your time and shows up—on time—for *all* appointments.

Let's take a step back from the canvas for a moment and admire this truly exciting portrait we have painted together. Imagine if your patients—all of them, every single one of them—

... paid on time

... appreciated everything you and your team do

... understood the proper role of insurance and paying for treatment

... referred other new Ideal Patients to your practice

... trusted the treatment presented and accepted all of it

... were educated as to the value of dentistry

... and respected your time and the time of everyone else in your office

Take a bow—for you have truly painted a masterpiece!

When I go through this exercise with my clients, they simply cannot believe that their patients could ever meet this ideal standard. Your patients can and will meet this ideal standard, so let's talk for a few moments about exactly how to make that happen.

> **FIRST, MEET WITH YOUR TEAM AND TELL THEM THAT YOUR OFFICE IS ONLY GOING TO TREAT IDEAL PATIENTS FROM NOW ON. GET AN AGREEMENT WITH YOUR TEAM AS TO WHAT THE IDEAL PATIENT LOOKS LIKE.**

First, meet with your team and tell them that your office is only going to treat Ideal Patients from now on. Get an agreement with your team as to what the Ideal Patient looks like. In other words, show them the word portrait that you have just painted, and explain that this is the kind of patient that you are going to treat from now on.

Let them know that transforming your patients from their current situations to a place where they are all Ideal Patients will take at least six months, and it must be and will be an ongoing commitment on your part and on the part of every member of your team.

Next, you want to set up a plan for implementing this new process. If you've put into place everything we've discussed in Chapters 3 through 7, your practice will now be set up to take on new projects like this. That's because you have created accountability by position. Everybody in your office knows exactly what he or she is supposed to do, how, and why. Implementation of this Ideal Patient program works this way: Everyone in your office is responsible for re-educating patients about his or her aspect of the practice.

What exactly does that mean? Let's start with your appointment coordinator. Your appointment coordinator now has the responsibility of re-educating patients about the fact that appointments are to be kept and arrived at on time. The people in charge of the finances in your office are to re-educate existing patients about new agreements regarding finances. People in charge of patient education and sales are to re-educate existing patients about new agreements in this area. It's not about making your patients wrong for what's happened in the past. Instead, it's about you, through your team, taking responsibility for what has happened in the past, and setting new standards for the future.

Your team members will be telling your patients essentially the following: "Up until now, we ran our office one way. We've now decided to make some upgrades to our practice, to make the practice better for everyone. We are now having everyone in our office take specific responsibilities for different areas of our practice, and it's going to be great for you. This way, we can provide you with the absolute best experience in our office."

Then your people will explain that arriving late, paying late, or all the other luxuries in which patients previously have been free to indulge are no longer acceptable. Those are, in fact, the magic words that will issue from your team's mouths over and over and over, until your patients have been re-educated: "It's no longer acceptable to… "

Your team members have to speak courteously and calmly to your patients, but they have to set these limits. I spend an enormous amount of time with my clients, working with every single member of their teams, to train them in this incredibly important task of reeducating patients. Together, we role-play the specific situations that occur, go over the most effective language to use, and determine how best to handle the various levels of problem situations their patients present.

IT'S NOT THE EASIEST THING IN THE WORLD TO RETRAIN PATIENTS, AND MANY UNIQUE SITUATIONS ARISE.

The dentists and their team members call me, sometimes twice and three times a day, as they're implementing this Ideal Patient approach. It's not the easiest thing in the world to retrain patients, and many unique situations arise. So it truly is up to the dentist to be committed to implementing this process throughout the office, with every patient, and I work very hard with my clients to get them through this often challenging transition period.

Sustained implementation of the Ideal Patient approach will exist only if every morning team meeting is dedicated to troubleshooting. Everybody's going to have situations that they want to discuss, and you've got to be prepared to talk about these things with your team members every single morning. The form of the morning meeting is

"YTT"—Yesterday Today Tomorrow. In other words, your team will first talk about what happened yesterday, then discuss what you're expecting today, and then talk a little bit about where things are headed tomorrow and in the future with the Ideal Patient program.

You can expect the first ninety days to be challenging, because everyone is going to be learning new roles—you, your team, and your patients. Your team will be counting on you to supervise this process. You can also count on the fact that patients will test you, push back against this new process, and challenge you. Under no circumstances should you waver. This is an intense period, but one that produces the most phenomenal results—Ideal Patients who resemble in every way the portrait we painted earlier. Again, someone has to be in control of your practice. It's either going to be you, or it's going to be the patients. If it's you, and if you are essentially forcing your patients to conform to this higher standard, a few of them may go away. Those are the ones who were probably the hardest to deal with: the most disruptive ones due to their lateness, cancellations, or broken appointments and the ones who were the least likely to pay. Good riddance to them.

It takes some courage for a dentist to say, "I want to serve only patients who resemble the portrait I created in my mind of the Ideal Patient." But I'm sure you agree with me that if you hold your current patients to these higher standards and thus transform them into Ideal Patients, everything will improve. You've now become the Ideal Dentist. Your team has become the Ideal Team. Your patients have attained the status of Ideal Patients. Once again, these changes will be reflected in your own level of enjoyment and serenity… and in your bottom line.

Another important subject to discuss, when it comes to improving your relationships with your patients, is the concept of control. Everybody feels more comfortable when they are in control of the situation. Control is one of the biggest results that my clients enjoy as a result of our work together—and in most cases, they didn't even know to ask for it. When I ask my clients what they want out of our work together, they always say they want to make more money. Many of them say that they want to experience less frustration in their work. But seldom does a client ask for an increase in a sense of control of his or her life. And yet this is a natural by-product of the kind of work that I do with my clients.

My clients quickly learn that control is worth more than money, because you can create anything you choose, including more money, when you're in control. So I want to show you a new way to achieve a sense of control in your relationships with your patients, because when you control the situation, things will go much better for everyone.

There are two kinds of control. First, there's the type of control that I don't advocate. This is the kind of dictatorial control that you see in socialistic or totalitarian governments, where one person or a small group of people possesses all the power, to the detriment of everyone else in society. Instead, I'm talking about the kind of healthy control that can be best illustrated by the traffic signals you see—and follow—every day. Traffic signals provide a type of control that is automatic, unquestioned, and honored, because if we fail to honor those signals, there are natural built-in consequences. We risk accidents, injuries, or citations from police, who always happen to be right there the "one time" we speed through the yellow light.

MY CLIENTS QUICKLY LEARN THAT CONTROL IS WORTH MORE THAN MONEY, BECAUSE YOU CAN CREATE ANYTHING YOU CHOOSE, INCLUDING MORE MONEY, WHEN YOU'RE IN CONTROL.

The kind of control exemplified by traffic signals provides a win-win situation for everyone. We all get to arrive at our destinations safely and with a minimum of tension and frustration.

You can think of what's going to follow in this chapter as a means of providing traffic signals for your patients. Most of the time, when I come into a client's office for the first time, no one is in control. Everything just sort of happens chaotically. The doctor rushes from room to room. The front desk is scrambling to keep up with the latest crisis. Patients arrive and pay for treatment either late or not at all. This is no way to run a traffic system—and it's no way to run an office!

So the question becomes how do we gain good control—the kind of automatic, unquestioned control that traffic signals provide—with your current patients, who, after all, have essentially been "trained" to contribute to the chaos in your practice? How do we get them on board with the idea that we are moving from chaos to healthy control and that your office is going to control its own destiny, perhaps for the first time?

Let's start with some great news. Even the dentists most uncomfortable at presenting cases are transformed into *powerhouses* when they implement the suggestions I've offered you in Chapters 3 through 7 of this book. Now they've got an entire office backing them up. They're practicing the kind of dentistry they want to practice, in a calm, harmonious, extremely lucrative environment. They realize that they've finally become the dentists they've always wanted to be.

The analogy that I like to share with my clients is that of Michelangelo's David. Michelangelo famously said that his job was to free the sculpture from the marble that surrounded it. In other words, by chipping away at the extraneous pieces that should not have been there, he arrived at the perfect sculpture, and his sculptures have touched the hearts of viewers for more than five hundred years.

Similarly, when you chip away at all the unnecessary limitations that inhibit your ability to practice dentistry at the highest level, the real you—the Michelangelo's David trapped in the marble—emerges. How can you *not* perform a thousand times better when you are no longer trapped by the thinking patterns and behaviors that held back the real you? This process will chip away at everything that doesn't belong, leaving you with the ability to be the caring, committed, and amazingly successful dentist you deserve to be.

Okay, Dr. Powerhouse. Let's talk about three transformations that will take place in you simply as a result of putting into practice everything that we've talked about in Chapters 3 through 7. These three transformations focus on the way you relate to your patients.

1. The First Transformation Means Moving from Doubt to Certainty.

Dentists who are afraid to present cases to their patients, out of fear of rejection or whatever other reason, convey a sense of doubt and uncertainty to their patients. It's a little like the guy who steps up to the craps table in the casino with a scared look in his eyes. He takes everybody down. The casino term is "scared money," and scared money never wins. The one thing that your patients, your team, and your family all want from you is a sense of certainty.

Nobody wants to sense doubt in a medical professional. Think about it—your patients are simply not in a position to determine whether you are the world's greatest dental practitioner or just an average Joe. But they sure can tell whether you convey a sense of doubt or certainty, and if they sense your doubt, their own fears will multiply when they see you holding a handpiece. By implementing the procedures we've talked about in the preceding chapters, you will come across as the absolute embodiment of certainty. Your patients will respond to you more positively, because you are giving them what they most desire—a sense that they are in good hands.

2. The Second Transformation is Moving from Survival to Caring.

Most dentists have an attitude of simply surviving—of getting through the day. They see their day as a series of unpleasant situations and crises that require their attention, instead of seeing their day as an opportunity to serve others, bring the highest level of dental care to their patients, and, not so coincidentally, make really great money in the process. The problem is that if you are focused on survival, you are focused on you.

If you don't think a patient can sense that aura of desperation that a person in survival mode invariably exudes, you're fooling yourself. They can tell. It's always shocking to a patient to see a dentist who is harried, harassed, and otherwise unhappy. After all, the patient knows that a dentist is an individual who runs his own shop, who makes a lot of money, and who lives a very nice lifestyle. What exactly do you have to complain about, the patient wonders, as he or she sees you heading into the hygienist's room.

Patients can smell fear. If you are operating in survival mode, you are thinking first, last, and always about you. The alternative, of course, is to think about the patient. If you don't have any worries, if your team is working with you and not against you, if everyone from the hygienist to the appointment coordinator to the treatment coordinator to the re-care coordinator to your assistant knows exactly what his or her job is and is doing it beautifully, you can focus all of your energy on the patient. You can afford to care, because you now have the emotional energy to devote to thinking about the needs of your patient instead of thinking about your own situation. The move from survival to caring is key if you want your patients to believe that you are in control of the situation.

YOU CAN AFFORD TO CARE, BECAUSE YOU NOW HAVE THE EMOTIONAL ENERGY TO DEVOTE TO THINKING ABOUT THE NEEDS OF YOUR PATIENT INSTEAD OF THINKING ABOUT YOUR OWN SITUATION.

3. The Third and Final Transformation is From Blaming Others to Recognizing That You Can Cause Things to Go Right.

Most people, even most successful people, go through their lives thinking of themselves as victims. The world is doing it to me, they sob. Poor, poor, pitiful me. I'm such a victim. Everything conspires against me. I can't get anything right. We all know people like that, sometimes we all think this way, often without realizing it.

The simple fact is that nobody likes a person with a victim mentality, and again, this is just as hard to hide as that survival mode we were talking about a moment ago. The fact is that you are not a victim. You may have created the sense of chaos in your thinking and in your dental practice. The unpleasant reality that people who want to be highly successful have to face is that they are the authors of their own lives. Yes, tragedy happens in life, but I'm not talking about tragedy. I'm talking about the situation that is bound to occur when a dentist manages a practice based on his emotions, based on his financial crises, and based on anything other than the kind of principles we are talking about in this book.

The dentists I work with learn to take responsibility for the fact that they helped create the situation in which they have found themselves. They caused it. Once they realize they caused it, once they free themselves from the blame game, they realize they have the same amount of power with which to cure these problems. And with the ideas that we've been talking about in this book, they have a method for curing those problems, and they have a method for running their office in a way that truly benefits everyone—themselves, their teams, their patients, and their families. So it's essential for a successful individual, or an individual who wants to achieve a high level of success, to let go of the finger-pointing mentality, to begin to recognize that we are indeed the authors of our lives and begin to take action to remedy the past and chart a course for a brighter future.

Those are the three Cs that your patients want you to display: they want to see you as certain, as caring, and as causative. These three Cs lead to the fourth and most important C of all—control. If you don't control your practice, your patients will, by showing up and paying whenever they feel like it, instead of adhering to agreements into which you cause them to enter.

To summarize what we've discussed in this chapter, you have the right to transform your current patients into Ideal Patients. You've earned this right because you've transformed your office into the Ideal Office, and you've transformed yourself into the Ideal Dentist! We concentrated in this chapter on your current patients. Now, how do you attract only Ideal New Patients to your practice? That's the subject of Chapter 9.

Take Your Practice to the NextLevel:

1. Now that your office is running in an ideal manner, you're entitled to be seeing only Ideal Patients.

2. Create your own concept of the Ideal Patient. Then, work with your team to transform your current patients into the Ideal Patients you would prefer to treat.

    Right now, name five of your favorite patients. What are their qualities and attributes? What makes them different from your least favorite patients? Identifying the traits you're seeking—and the traits you're keen to avoid—will help you know what to look for as you make a composite of your Ideal Patient.

3. An Ideal Patient pays on time, appreciates everything you and your team do, understands the proper role of insurance and paying for treatment, refers other Ideal Patients to your practice, trusts the treatment presented and accepts all of it, is educated as to the value of dentistry, and respects your time and the time of everyone else in your office. Ideal Patients are the type of patient you deserve.

    To add to your roster of Ideal Patients, call your current top five patients and tell them how happy you are to have their business. Then ask if they know anyone like them whom they would be willing to refer to you. You might also suggest that they give you names and numbers of people so that you can call them yourself.

Chapter 9

Getting Off the
New Patient Treadmill

MOST DENTISTS THINK that new patients are the lifeblood of their practice, responsible for maintaining and increasing the success and cash flow of the practice. In fact, new patients typically consume far more energy and resources than most dentists realize. These dentists churn through the maximum number of new patients every month in order to maintain cash flow and the growth of their practices. Yet this approach doesn't provide a very high return on investment. Most of the new patients will cycle through the practice and be gone within a year, leaving behind a wake of diagnostic work performed leading to cases not presented, or cases inserted and not paid for. Either way, relying on new patients to shore up a dental practice is a recipe for disaster. Perhaps one dentist in a thousand realizes this.

I want to give you a new way to think about new patients, a new way to integrate them into your system, and a method for transforming these individuals into the Ideal Patients whom we discussed in the previous chapter. The system I am going to share with you for integrating new patients into your practice will make you so much money, saving you up to a week of non-productive chair time per month and greatly reducing stress and rejection, that you will scarcely believe it. One client of mine averaged just four new patients a month in the first three months of implementing this system and increased his monthly gross income by $75,000—by the third month.

NEW PATIENTS TYPICALLY CONSUME FAR MORE ENERGY AND RESOURCES THAN MOST DENTISTS REALIZE.

Keep in mind that your new patient, one in which you are investing a great deal of effort and resources, is most likely some other dentist's problem ex-patient. Most dentists are just happy to have a new warm body in the reception area. Yet that warm body might have been dismissed from someone else's practice for broken or cancelled appointments or simply may have caused upheaval due to chaotic, angry, or unpleasant behavior. Most dentists never ask themselves the simple question, "Why does this person need a new dentist?" That's because most dentists are approaching life from a survival mindset, and when you're thinking in terms of survival, any new patient, no matter how ornery or slow to pay, will do.

Some people are dissatisfied with life in general, not just with dentists, and they essentially travel from dentist to dentist in search of some seemingly unattainable ideal, failing to respect the quality of treatment the dentist offers, the time of the dentist, hygienist, or the rest of the team, or the dentist's legitimate right to be compensated in full and on time for services rendered.

There are few dental virgins out there. Just about every adult in our society has had treatment from some dentist or other, so when we discuss new patients, we're not really talking about a completely "new" human being. We're just talking about someone who is new to your office. And chances are that if your office handles them in the same way they've been handled by other dental offices, that individual is going to wreak just as much damage on your bottom line, your happiness, and your team's well-being as he or she has caused to your colleagues. These people are drains on time, money, and emotions, and you have the responsibility—and the *right*—to refuse to allow them to cause you grief.

THERE ARE FEW DENTAL VIRGINS OUT THERE.

When you have put into practice the suggestions I have shared with you, the simple fact is that you won't have a lot of time left over for new patients. Whenever I perform a chart audit, I see millions of dollars in treatment that could be provided, had the dentist only possessed the courage—and the system—to turn that necessary dental work into treatment closed, inserted, and paid for. Most dentists collect less than a hundred percent for the work they have performed, especially as a percentage of the work their current patients need, so they rely far too heavily on churning new patients through the office. Unfortunately, these dentists are as unlikely to present and close cases to new patients as they are to existing patients.

The psychological explanation is very straightforward. It's harder to close a case with a new patient, because the dentist hasn't yet earned the trust of that patient. As a result, many dentists don't even bother trying to present or close complex cases to new patients. They'll settle for getting some work—a few fillings, perhaps—but they aren't providing the patient with the care that patient really needs. This hurts the patient, who needs comprehensive care, and it hurts the dental practice, because you don't get to serve the patient to the fullest and thus maximize your income.

Let's go a little deeper into the problems that new patients present to a dental practice. I performed a study which revealed that new patients on average accept only seventeen percent of the treatment presented, and only thirty-eight percent of new patients are retained as patients after the first year. My survey also indicated that half of their new patients were in fact the exact kind of people they did not want in their offices—individuals who left another dentist owing money, claiming to have been "treated poorly." Why would you allow these people free entry into your office without any sort of qualification? You are basically giving them a driver's license without even making them take a road test! What kind of driving am I talking about? Driving you crazy!

The other problem about new patients coming from other dentists' offices is that they assume that your office runs just as inefficiently as the dental and medical offices they have visited in the past. In other words, their prior dental and medical practitioners essentially trained them to be mediocre patients. How did those dentists and other medical professionals train these patients poorly? Think about your own experience when you go see a doctor. Chances are, you were seen late and forced to wait, regardless of the havoc this played with your schedule. This essentially "trained" you to believe that since the doctor didn't respect your time, you were under no obligation to respect his. In those other offices, the patients were allowed to change appointments at will, confounding the ability of the office to get things done on time.

Another way in which medical doctors "create" problem patients relates to payment. A doctor creates value in the mind of the patient when he shows just how much the work he'll perform is *worth* to the patient. Yet most doctors never share with their patients the sense that their work is worth more than the $20 co-pay. Perhaps the doctor is performing services worth $2,000—but if the doctor doesn't tell the patient, how will the patient know?

Is a doctor's training and experience worth only twenty bucks to a patient? The answer is yes, unless and until the doctor trains the patient to think otherwise. Patients think the doctor is "worth" only the amount of their co-pay. That's training a patient to disrespect the doctor. And that disrespectful attitude toward the doctor's time and treatment spills over into the way that patient will feel about you, his dentist.

Most medical offices, and most dental offices, too, for that matter, fail to give the patients a sense of love and appreciation—what I call the Ritz-Carlton effect. When you walk into a Ritz-Carlton lobby, you're treated like you're a billionaire unless and until you choose to inform them otherwise! You're greeted with a smile and you are made to feel respected and special. Ritz-Carlton spares no expense creating that warm and fuzzy feeling, and its millions of guests don't mind paying more for the sense of trust and respect they enjoy every time they arrive. But do patients in most doctors' and dentists' offices get a warm and fuzzy feeling? Where is the love? Nowhere. And patients reciprocate the feeling that they aren't important by treating your time with disrespect. That's why patients feel so free to cancel appointments at the last minute, show up late, or fail to show up at all. They sense that you don't care about them, so why should they care about you?

Not only do most health care providers fail to make the patient feel special, *they also provide little to no patient education, which is just as bad.* Unfortunately, most dentists and doctors are focused primarily on increasing volume in order to meet their own financial survival needs, instead of coming from a place of caring for each individual patient. They may *want* to give each patient tender loving care, but they believe that they simply don't have time to do so. They're on a survival treadmill, and it only spins faster and faster.

These harried dentists don't see the value of creating a patient education system because they don't see how it puts cash in their pockets right away. By now, you've seen that patient education is the missing link between where you are financially and where you want to be. Yet patients in those offices are exposed only to solutions, without a clear explanation in lay person's terms of the problems that need to be treated. They are given no education as to why the proposed care is vital—*and worth every dollar*. To top it off, these other offices have failed to enter into agreements with the patients—agreements that cover the nature of the treatment, the time frame for the treatment, and the method and timing of payment.

In short, all of your colleagues—doctors *and* dentists— are working overtime to train your potential new patients to be bad patients. Obviously, this is simply not going to work in the new kind of system that you are implementing. So I'd like to share with you now the four key elements in eliminating new patient inefficiency.

First, establish the team as the patient's trusted advisor. Here comes the Ritz-Carlton warm and fuzzy. Here comes the love. Here comes your team, establishing themselves not just as a drill, fill, and bill operation, but as the most caring group of dental professionals your patient has ever encountered. It's your responsibility to institute a method by which your team is established quickly in the mind of the patient as the most trusted advisor the patient will ever need with regard to dental care. The system we have spoken about does this automatically. The patient clearly understands who is leading whom. This causes him or her to listen to you differently, as a trusted advisor.

The second element in eliminating new patient inefficiency is for you and the rest of your team to be aware of your new patient's motivating values. In other words, what do they want out of their relationship with your dental practice? If you don't ask, you'll never know, and if you don't know, the chances are slim that you'll be able to meet their expectations and desires. You'll base your thinking on assumptions instead of the patient's reality. How can you uncover a patient's motivating values? During the trust exam, learn where your patient is in life. Ask the simple question, "Tell me about yourself."

Listen carefully for upcoming life events that trigger the desire for people to look and feel healthier and more attractive. Life events such as college reunions, "odometer" birthdays (turning 30, 40, 50, etc.), getting married, or getting divorced are enormous incentives to people to maintain and enhance their health and appearance. Find out if such events are on your new patients' horizons. And if so, don't be afraid to suggest the care or cosmetic work that will allow them to look and feel their best.

> **WHAT DO THEY WANT OUT OF THEIR RELATIONSHIP WITH YOUR DENTAL PRACTICE? IF YOU DON'T ASK, YOU'LL NEVER KNOW, AND IF YOU DON'T KNOW, THE CHANCES ARE SLIM THAT YOU'LL BE ABLE TO MEET THEIR EXPECTATIONS AND DESIRES.**

The third element in eliminating new patient inefficiency is to know the patient's fears and concerns. Just about everybody who walks into a dental office is afraid of something. Maybe it's the sound of the drill. Maybe it's the pain they associate with dentistry. Maybe it's the needle. Maybe it's paying for the dental treatment. Maybe it's just being there. But it's fair to say that a hundred percent of the patients who enter your office bring with them some sort of fear. It's your job and the job of your team to determine exactly what each new patient's specific fears and concerns are, so that you can address those fears and concerns. Again, if you don't ask, they won't tell. And if they don't tell you what they're afraid of, they will skip appointments and break agreements rather than face their fears.

Let's take an extra moment to talk about dealing with each patient's fears. Dentists are certainly aware in a general way that most dental patients experience fear when they come in for treatment. Yet most dentists don't take the time to discern exactly what each specific patient's fears are. When the patient knows that you know the precise nature of her fears, she will feel safer. Fear will loosen its tight grip on her. She'll feel that you and she are in partnership to overcome her fears—it's two against one, you and the patient against the patient's fear. And the two of you, together, will vanquish that fear every time. Do you see the kind of loyalty that such an act of caring on your part creates?

WITH NEW PATIENTS, YOU WANT TO TAKE POSITIVE, HEALTHY CONTROL FROM THE VERY START.

More than any other factor, fear keeps people from showing up for their appointments. If a patient doesn't want to show up for treatment or pay for treatment, take the time to go back to their motivating factors and comfort them on their fears. "Oh, you don't want to pay that bill? Remember we talked about how you didn't want to lose your teeth, and we talked about how we comforted you by numbing you before we numbed you."

The fourth and final element in eliminating new patient inefficiency is that you've got to take time up front to educate the patient on how to participate in your practice. Remember that in the last chapter we talked about the sense of control that emerges from the processes you've instituted in your office that we've outlined in this book. With new patients, you want to take positive, healthy control *from the very start.* Taking control means letting the patient know that there is a certain way to be a patient in this office, and it's different from the ways that patients are patients in the offices of other dentists and doctors.

Now let's talk about how to institute these different procedures.

The first thing to realize is that there are two types of patients. There are those who are willing to be coached by you and your team to become the Ideal Patients we discussed in the previous chapter. And then there are those who are more than willing to suck the life out of you as they sucked the life out of previous dentists who sought unsuccessfully to treat them and never even got paid for their troubles with these people. I think it's clear by now that the typical new patient, trained to be a poor patient by previous dental and medical practitioners, is the last person you ever want to set foot in your office. So the question becomes, how do you find those patients who are willing to be coached to meet the standards of your office? What steps are necessary in order to make the new patients you do accept career-long Ideal Patients for you and your team?

The first thing you want to figure out is just how many patients you are willing to see and also can fit in after all the new production you have created by implementing the steps I've outlined for you in this book. Again, you will find you have very little open time for new patients, so you no longer have to worry about where that constant stream of new patients will come from.

Getting off the new patient treadmill terrifies many dentists. They wonder how they'll survive financially if they aren't churning countless newbies through the practice. And yet, whenever I meet with a new client, I go into his or her software, to analyze the ratio of "treatment presented" to "treatment accepted and paid for." (Of course, I can do this only if treatment plans are entered into the system.) As I mentioned earlier, most dentists are leaving millions of dollars in the cabinets of their chartrooms. So you don't need a gazillion new patients if you're simply providing your *current* patients with the level of comprehensive care we've discussed earlier in this book. The simple fact is that if you offer your current patients the dentistry they need, *you'll never run out of work.*

GETTING OFF THE NEW PATIENT TREADMILL TERRIFIES MANY DENTISTS.

A metaphor I share with my clients is the painting and repainting of the George Washington Bridge. It takes four years to paint the entire bridge, and by the time the painters have completed the task, it's time to start over! Similarly, it will take you years to catch up with the decay and disease in your *current* patients' mouths, and by the time you finish that Herculean task, it'll be time to start over, because those current patients' dental health will worsen, for various reasons. The painters on the George Washington Bridge don't have to worry about finding new bridges to paint. And you won't have to worry about finding new patients, either. Take proper care of the people you already serve, and there will be very few free hours in your practice.

If you accept that logic, then the next question is this: How many new patients do you need in order to fill the (very small) gap in your schedule? Usually, my two-doctor practices see about fifteen new patients per month. This amount translates into the traditional amount of attrition patients who leave the practice due to moving, passing away, or other reasons. After my two dentist- practices have scheduled in their fifteenth new patient in any given month, the appointment coordinator books the next new patients into the next month so as not to bog down the system.

The appointment coordinator also is careful to schedule these new patients at designated times that make sense for the practice and for the patient. A time that works for the practice means not scheduling a new patient during peak times—just one new patient a day, maximum. If you're working sixteen days a month, like most of my clients, and you're seeing only fifteen new patients a month, you don't need to see more than one new patient a day. This also allows you to interact with each new patient with a degree of interest and friendliness that simply isn't possible for dentists who are churning the largest possible number of new patients through their schedules.

Let's assume that your practice currently welcomes forty new patients a month. The approach I've just outlined for you, in which you'll be seeing just fifteen new patients a month, saves you twenty-five patient visits, which equals twenty-five hours of your valuable time. This nets your practice twenty-five hugely productive hours to do work for your current patients, work that is already closed and paid for. What would you rather do, sell yourself to twenty-five strangers, most of whom won't be with your practice a year from now, or use that time to perform the kind of interesting and lucrative dentistry that you enjoy the most?

We're also limiting your new patients to the kinds of patients you really want to add to your practice. Keep in mind that we don't allow just any potential new patient to walk in the door and drive you and your team crazy. Instead, I teach my clients to set up a gatekeeper system. First, there is a telephone interview process by which the treatment coordinator, working in a quiet setting off the floor, is able to screen out those individuals who simply do not meet with the standards of the practice. These are the people who may owe money to their previous practitioners, can't pay, won't pay, rely too heavily on insurance, or are not interested in comprehensive and preventative care. These people have no right to your time and expertise.

If the potential new patient gets past that phone call (and most, but not all, do), an appointment is made for that potential new patient to meet with the treatment coordinator. In other words, before the new patient sees a hygienist, gets x-rays, or, above all, meets with the dentist, that new patient must first meet with the treatment coordinator for thirty minutes.

During this first session, the treatment coordinator will

further qualify the patient as to his or her ability to meet the financial expectations of the practice, then educate the patient as to the nature of the practice and the fact that *things work differently here.* My clients' treatment coordinators ask the specific questions that I have determined are the most effective at drawing out and addressing up front all their concerns, motivations, and fears. After the treatment coordinator has gone through that very thorough interview process with the new patient, she then gives the new patient an office tour. This is unlike any process that any patient experiences in any other office.

Some of my clients express a concern over whether their patients will really want to talk about their lives. Who has time for that in today's busy world? The simple reality is that people love to talk about themselves, and now you are providing them with the most valuable thing that most human beings crave: a willing ear. You create a huge bond of trust with your patients when you just simply listen to them talk about their lives, their past dental experiences, their fears, their financial issues. Your patients will never forget the fact that your office took the time to get to know them as people, to forge a bond of shared humanity, instead of looking at them strictly as a source of revenue and work.

THE SIMPLE REALITY IS THAT PEOPLE LOVE TO TALK ABOUT THEMSELVES, AND NOW YOU ARE PROVIDING THEM WITH THE MOST VALUABLE THING THAT MOST HUMAN BEINGS CRAVE: A WILLING EAR.

My clients also wonder exactly how many new patients they will be rejecting as a result of putting in these practices. It isn't many—it may just be one in fifty or even one in a hundred. More important, having this "gatekeeper" system in effect trains your new patients to respect the way things work in your office. Your new patients will now learn that they must show up on time. Since the office is a "zero-balance office," they learn that they will not be permitted to leave work unpaid for. Your office insists on making agreements with regard to appointments, financing, and other important matters. Your team tells the patient, "Please don't make the appointment unless you're sure you're going to show up. We really value appointments around here., so don't schedule an appointment you know you can't make. Dr. So-And-So is a stickler for patients showing up for their appointments on time."

It's extremely powerful to teach your patients that *your office is different*. The bottom line: You've established a different standard about the value of your own time inside your practice. And your patients will admire and respect you for having done so. When you've got a policy of explaining the "rules of the road" at your practice, you'll cut down enormously on stress and heartache for you and your team, and you'll weed out those individuals who will be nothing but serious trouble down the road. Most patients who might not have conformed in the past to these sorts of guidelines will do so for you and your team, because you're showing them the "bigger picture" as to how your office works. This allows them to see how they fit into your practice, instead of letting them decide how to fit your practice into their (often chaotic) lives.

Once the patient has passed the "test" of meeting with the treatment coordinator for thirty minutes in the treatment room, has been qualified financially, and has been educated as to the nature of the practice, only *then* will the patient proceed to the final round: meeting the dentist.

On the initial meeting with the client, the dentist performs the "trust exam" I mentioned earlier. I use this term because you are seeking, in this examination, to establish trust between you and the patient. Get connected with the patient. Say to him or her, "Tell me about yourself." Listen for common connectors—do they have children, do they live in the same town as you, where are they from—all the sort of humanizing facts that link us together in the common human experience. Also ask, "What would you like to know about me as your doctor?" Tell them where you went to dental school. Tell them how many kids you have. Tell them the name of your dog. In other words, you're trying to humanize yourself so that you're not some sort of robotic dental practitioner with no heart, no soul, and not an ounce of caring for the patient. It is important that you get to know the patient as a person before you're in the back being a clinician. This also helps to eliminate the two obsessive thoughts plaguing the new patient as they sit in the chair: Is this going to hurt me? And how much is it going to cost?

Once you have established your own humanity and trustworthiness, explain what will happen on this visit. Remember that you are constantly increasing the patient's trust when you show yourself to be in control in a courteous and kind way—and also when you eliminate the unknown.

You can dissolve just about any fear by reducing or taking away the oppressive element of the unknown.

Right now you might be thinking to yourself, "I don't have time to have all these conversations with new patients. I'm busy!" I have no doubt that you're busy, and that's why I suggest that you need spend only five minutes in this trust-building phase of the conversation. It doesn't take long, and the results will pay off tenfold.

After you've accomplished a sense of connectedness with your patient, instruct your hygienist to spend the next fifteen minutes doing x-rays. Then have the hygienist perform the intraoral tour of the mouth. Follow that by ten minutes of educating your patient, familiarizing them with what they need.

I like to tell my clients, "You've got to get in their heads before you can get in their mouths." By now, your patient will have been at the office for at least an hour and will thoroughly understand the nature of your practice and exactly *what is expected of him or her*.

Let's analyze what it takes to get a patient to trust you. First, you're establishing that bond of caring by spending five minutes just chatting about raising your kids, discovering that you both grew up in Scottsdale, or how much you love golf. Those first five minutes with the patient are the most valuable "real estate" in your portfolio. You're building on the bond of trust that the treatment coordinator, representing you and your practice, just spent half an hour creating. Your patient has never been treated like this anywhere—with the possible exception of the Ritz-Carlton.

To summarize:

Gary Kadi's New Patient Protocol

1. Phone interview with treatment coordinator.

2. In-Office interview with treatment coordinator.

3. "Trust Exam" with Dentist.

4. Tour of office with treatment coordinator.

5. Hygienist performs X-Rays.

6. Hygienist performs intraoral "Tour of the Mouth" and provides 10-Minute patient education to build their awareness of what was found.

7. Dentist comes into the room and confirms what the hygienist found with the intraoral camera.

8. Hygienist completes cleaning (if advanced care is not needed) and sets 6-month recare appointment.

9. Treatment coordinator explains care, handles financing, and schedules any dental work before closing the case.

10. Work is performed.

11. Patient enters re-care system.

You now have a clear sense of how my clients welcome appropriate new patients into their practices—and screen out all the rest. The last point I want to share with you in this chapter is that it is absolutely vital to schedule a patient into the re-care system. This is a huge bleeding point for most dental practices: they get new patients in the door, the patients get work done, and then the dentist never sees them again. So you'll be applying the NextLevel methodology of getting and keeping your new patients in the re-care system, using the same suggestions you found earlier in this book with your current patients.

In the beginning of the chapter, I made the assertion that new patients tend to have the exact opposite effect on dental practices than what most dentists think. Dentists typically assume that new patients equal new cash flow, whereas the reality is that for most dentists, new patients can equal new heartache. By now, you've retrained your team. You've retrained yourself in many important ways. You've retrained your current patients to turn them into Ideal Patients. And now you know how to train new patients to become the sort of ideal patients that you—and your practice—deserve.

NOW YOU KNOW HOW TO TRAIN NEW PATIENTS TO BECOME THE SORT OF IDEAL PATIENTS THAT YOU—AND YOUR PRACTICE—DESERVE.

If you think about the suggestions we've offered in this book as comprehensive care for the dental practice, you'll notice that there are no longer any bleeding points. We have a completely healthy situation, replacing the chaos, dysfunction, and red ink that might have existed previously.

Now that you have a clear picture of how to run your dental practice on these terms, I'd like to share with you a vision of what your dental practice will be like when all of this is implemented. You'll find that vision at the heart of our next and final chapter.

Take Your Practice to the NextLevel:

1. New patients typically consume far more energy and resources than most dentists realize.

2. No patient can cause you heartache without your permission. When your patient is aggravated or ticked off, ask them why they are so angry. Then ask if they are wiling to have a conversation with you about why they're mad. Be warned—some patients may be more interested in remaining ticked off than actually solving the problem. Just remember: if you continue to step over bad behavior, they will continue to behave badly.

3. When you get a new patient, you must try to understand their needs, desires, motivations, and fears. Learn to listen to what the patient is not saying. What does having the dental work provide for them? Who don't they get to be if their teeth remain like they are? For most people, not having nice teeth means the lack of a friendly smile or not looking attractive. The art of listening to your patients' unspoken sentiments is a great gift, one that will serve you well. To practice, converse with your spouse, listen both to what they're saying and what they're not.

4. Apply the New Patient Protocol to each new patient whom your office accepts. And don't forget to enroll your team. It takes a team to close a case.

Chapter 10

Attaining the NextLevel
in Your Practice

A S THE CREATOR OF the NextLevel Practice, I'm happiest when I get calls from clients with whom I worked a decade ago and they tell me that the systems we installed back then are still going strong and that the office is making huge amounts of money—with ease. Everyone's having a great time because they all—the dentist, the team members, and the patients—know their roles. The office runs smoothly, there's a waiting list of new patients stretching out for months, turnover is at a minimum, and they're constantly getting bombarded with calls and résumés from highly talented people who want to work there.

Why shouldn't you have the same kind of experience as my current and past clients? Why shouldn't you have an office that absolutely mints money for you, while providing the highest level of care for your patients? Why shouldn't you have a stress-free existence, a chaos-free office, a much bigger net worth, and a more serene home life? You're entitled to it. And you've seen in this book how to achieve it.

Sometimes my clients tell me, "I knew I needed to do a lot of these things before you came on board. But you showed me how to make these changes stick… and stick forever."

WHY SHOULDN'T YOU HAVE AN OFFICE THAT ABSOLUTELY MINTS MONEY FOR YOU, WHILE PROVIDING THE HIGHEST LEVEL OF CARE FOR YOUR PATIENTS?

Let's take a look at the three major shifts that occur when the NextLevel Practice System is installed. These three critical distinctions will separate you from the typical dentist. You'll be aware of these distinctions every day, your team will be aware of them, and your patients will be aware of them.

The first distinction: Most people perceive that dentists cause pain. Yet your patients experience the fact that you make them feel good. When was the last time you heard patients say, "I can't wait to go to the dentist"? It's not because you've got the latest LaserGuy 5000 office gear. It's because you and your team relate to your patients as human beings, maintaining the integrity of their dental health in an atmosphere of shared respect.

YOU AND YOUR TEAM RELATE TO YOUR PATIENTS AS HUMAN BEINGS, MAINTAINING THE INTEGRITY OF THEIR DENTAL HEALTH IN AN ATMOSPHERE OF SHARED RESPECT.

From the time your patients step into your reception area, they sense that they are in for something different. You take the time to get to know your patients on a personal level, and you allow them a little bit of insight into your life. They've come through the treatment coordinator's office, which allowed them to get to know you, your team, your accomplishments, your successful patients, and your office's community involvement. You've given your patients a sense that you're in calm, quiet control of a harmonious, thriving dental practice. You've shown them that you care. You've shown them that they matter to you, and that you want to make an important difference in their lives. Most dentists are perceived as causing pain. You make your patients feel good—emotionally and physically—about the outstanding dental care they are so fortunate to receive.

One of the frustrations for most dentists is their awareness of the patients' needs and their inability to get the patients to agree to have their needs met. Now you and your team can fulfill your desire to provide care and meet your patients' needs for treatment. Communication, not chaos, is the soul of your practice. Your team is happy, too. A common team comment in my clients' offices: "I love coming to work because I know I'm really helping people."

The second distinction is that patients perceive most dentists as commodities. You now provide an experience.

One of the most powerful trends in society today is the transformation of virtually all goods and services into commodities. The Internet allows us to shop easily for price, and we buy in an impersonal manner from websites, 800 numbers, or "big box" stores where we seldom see the same sales clerk twice. The world has become so price-sensitive that it's so hard for anyone to charge a premium and justify that higher price.

The "personal touch" is vanishing from our world, and the so- called service economy provides little to no service at all. But you're different. While other dentists provide dental service as a commodity, be it a crown, a filling, or a bridge, you provide an experience, thanks to the fact that you display your caring for your patients, you educate them, and you make them feel special and important from the time they enter the reception area.

The closest parallel to your dental practice is, remarkably enough, Starbucks. At Starbucks, the raw beans for one cup of coffee cost about three cents. To roast and package those beans costs about fifteen cents. The service involved in brewing a cup of coffee probably costs the company twenty-five cents—and that includes the cup, the ground rent, the utilities, the Starbucks' sign, and the smiling barista's salary and benefits. (Barista? What's a barista? Just a fancy word for coffeemaker.)

The experience of going to a Starbucks for that cup of coffee that costs the company around forty-three cents costs the coffee lover four dollars. You could get that same cup of coffee in a diner for a buck. Yet millions upon millions of discerning, price-sensitive consumers will stand in line to pay the extra three dollars, day after day, just for the experience of being at Starbucks.

Now let's compare the Starbucks' experience to getting some dental work done. Let's take the example of having a crown put in. The basic underlying commodity for a crown—the "coffee beans," if you will—is a few dollars' worth of porcelain. It costs the typical dental office about a hundred fifty dollars to make an impression and provide instructions to the lab. To seat a crown (the dental equivalent of brewing and pouring a cup of coffee, because it's a fairly standard procedure) costs a dental office about five hundred dollars. A regular dentist who permits himself to be viewed as a commodity can charge about eight hundred dollars for installing a crown.

YOUR PATIENT SENSES, ACCURATELY, THAT YOUR OFFICE IS A SPECIAL PLACE, NOT THE DENTAL EQUIVALENT OF THE DINER ON THE HIGHWAY.

What about you? You're Starbucks. Your patient senses, accurately, that your office is a special place, not the dental equivalent of the diner on the highway. Because you are providing an experience and not simply a commodity to your patient, you legitimately charge a thousand or more. People can and will pay a very high premium if they believe that they are being treated well, and that is exactly what you offer your patients.

People go to Starbucks—and willingly pay that three-dollar premium—because *they like the experience of being there.* Similarly, you provide an experience that patients cannot find in most other dental offices. You create value. You get insurance information before the patient comes in. You understand the patient by taking the time to get to know his motivating factors and fears. You visually unveil problems with the intraoral camera, instead of leaping to the solution. You have a treatment coordinator to explain the problem, the consequences, and the solution. You completely explain the patient's financial responsibility, the benefits of their insurance, and the total investment for their care. You know how to use third-party financing effectively to fit people's budgets. You take away the unknown by explaining the treatment in terms that minimize fear and add benefit. You deliver virtually pain-free treatment. You educate patients on how to maximize their investments through solid preventative care and its long-term health benefits.

It all adds up to this simple fact: *you're not a commodity.* Other dentists, unfortunately for them, their team members, and their bankbooks, are indistinguishable one from the other.

Finally, the third and last distinction: The welfare of your patients and their loyalty to you and your staff have now become first and foremost in your practice.

By installing the NextLevel Practice system, you will stand out from the rest of the crowd. Being limited by what insurance covers is no longer a concern. You have the freedom to address the needs of your entire patient base and the flexibility of insurance to assist in the patient's overall oral wellness.

Let's now see how these distinctions will determine the future of your practice.

As a result of instituting the procedures we've discussed, you come to work each day to lead a harmonious team whose members are just as interested in your success as they are in their own. They are all much happier, because they've got clear responsibilities, accountabilities, and incentives to help you grow your practice. Your income is predictable month-to-month, so you're no longer worried about making payroll or cashing your paychecks. And your income continues to explode year after year, so you have the financial freedom you've always sought.

Your team is happy because they're making more money than ever and more money than most of their peers. You're not bothered by that, because you've learned to view salary as an investment rather than an expense. The more dollars they make, the more hundreds of thousands of dollars you make. Your office is a harmonious place where people love to come to work and where your patients feel the difference.

Your patients are different, too. It wasn't always easy, but you led your team through that re-education experience for your existing patients, and you instituted procedures that practically guaranteed that the few new patients you have time to see are all Ideal Patients as well. Your patients truly appreciate everything that you and your team do for them, and they tell their friends about your practice. You've got a waiting list for new patients that stretches months into the future.

AND YOUR INCOME CONTINUES TO EXPLODE YEAR AFTER YEAR, SO YOU HAVE THE FINANCIAL FREEDOM YOU'VE ALWAYS SOUGHT.

And what about you? You're chairside eighty percent of the time, doing exactly the kind of dentistry that interests you the most. You're making more money than you ever dreamt possible. You don't have to sell, because your team sells on your behalf. You've established a new, higher level of integrity for yourself that has created in your team the kind of respect for you that you always desired. You are working far fewer hours and far fewer days, and you've either cut down or eliminated entirely nights and weekends.

Somehow everything goes more smoothly in your life— not just at work, but at home as well. That sense of control and harmony that you have instituted at the office now replicates itself in your home life. There's a very good chance that your family relationships are stronger, your ties to your mate are healthier, and you even get along better with your kids. When you don't have all those worries about money and team draining your energy, you've got a lot more time and energy for your family. Other people dream of having balance in their lives. You've achieved it.

Your colleagues and dental school classmates spend their nights and weekends chairside. You? You're poolside!

Best of all, you no longer have that horrible feeling of running faster and faster on a cash-flow treadmill. You no longer walk around with a couple of paychecks in your wallet that you can't cash because the cash flow simply won't permit you to do so. If you had any personal debt, you've long since paid it all off. You sleep better at night, and so do those around you.

YOUR COLLEAGUES AND DENTAL SCHOOL CLASSMATES SPEND THEIR NIGHTS AND WEEKENDS CHAIRSIDE. YOU? YOU'RE POOLSIDE!

I want to acknowledge you for being the kind of person who is willing to take their business and their life to something beyond the ordinary. Ordinary people do not look at anything beyond the day-to-day function of business. The fact that you took the time to read this book says a great deal about the kind of person you are. You're someone with a commitment to living an extraordinary life and having a business that provides value to the customers it serves. You're also serious about improving the lives of both your employees and your family. Congratulations!

I'm proud to say that I've helped many dentists achieve the vision put forth in this book. There are three options I'd like to leave you with today:

First, after reading this book, you may essentially decide to leave things the way they are in your practice. It may well be that few or perhaps none of the problems we've discussed in this book apply to your office, so you don't need to make any changes.

The second option is that you've come to realize that the ideas in this book would make a dramatic difference if applied to your practice. So you may want to share these ideas with your team members and begin to implement them without outside assistance.

The third choice is to contact me and set up a time to talk. I'm happy to have written a book that shares these ideas, helping many dentists increase their income, satisfaction level, and the functionality of their practice. But I am doubly privileged to work with dentists on a one-on-one basis to fully implement the system, watching as their practices reach levels of success they never imagined. I invite you to contact me at Gary@GaryKadi.com so we can discuss the ways in which I can help you take your dental practice to the next level. There really is no risk—I guarantee dollar-for-dollar results based on your investment.

Thank you for taking the time to read this book. I know how valuable the time of a dentist truly is, and I appreciate the respect you've given my ideas. My wish is that this marks the beginning of a long and successful relationship between the two of us. I'll look forward to hearing from you.